*Epidemiology, Nursing
and Healthcare*

Also by Anne Mulhall:

M. Hardey and A. Mulhall (1994) *Nursing Research: Theory & Practice*, Chapman & Hall, London

Epidemiology, Nursing and Healthcare

A New Perspective

ANNE MULHALL
BSc, MSc, PhD

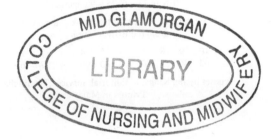

MACMILLAN

First published 1996 by
MACMILLAN PRESS LTD
Houndmills, Basingstoke, Hampshire RG21 6XS
and London
Companies and representatives
throughout the world

ISBN 0–333–62252–9 paperback

A catalogue record for this book is available
from the British Library.

10   9   8   7   6   5   4   3   2   1
05 04 03 02 01 00 99 98 97 96

Typeset by Ian Kingston Editorial Services, Nottingham
Printed in Malaysia

For Liam

CONTENTS

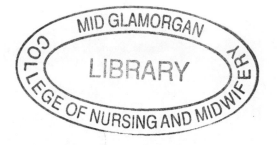

PREFACE

Firmly embedded within medicine, and adopting the paradigm[1] of the natural sciences, traditional epidemiology is ill equipped to contribute to a model of nursing[2] characterised by holism and naturalism. However, in an era when the planning, provision and evaluation of health services are increasingly fashioned on the basis of 'hard' statistics and 'objective' measures of need and quality, the discipline of epidemiology has gained new prominence. The restructuring of the health service and the emergence of the internal market have precipitated major changes in the philosophical and organisational character of the NHS. Quality assurance and evaluation programmes are being developed to maximise the effective and efficient delivery of care to patients, who have been transformed into consumers. Planning healthcare within this new environment demands a greater emphasis on the development of good information systems, widespread and effective health technology assessment, timely economic evaluations, and appropriate health need and health gain measures. Such initiatives and strategies are deemed vital if the targets outlined in *The Health of the Nation* (Department of Health, 1992a) are to be realised. Many of the methods traditionally used in epidemiological studies are providing the evidence to guide both research and organisational strategies in the new health service.

Within the last decade traditional epidemiology has broadened to assume two distinctive frames of reference. Historically located largely in the province of medicine, *clinical epidemiology* is a natural progression grounded in the roots of the parent discipline. Clinical epidemiology is concerned with the application of epidemiological concepts and principles at the micro-level of the clinical encounter. *Social epidemiology* considers the relationship between socio-economic factors and health. This area has generally been overlooked by hospital-based doctors and researchers, but is increasingly realised within the concepts of the new public health (Scott-Samuel, 1989) and the arguments that much of today's environment gratuitously damages people's health (Draper, 1991). This latter aspect is addressed in the new social epidemiology, which encompasses *popular epidemiology* – a synthesis of political

---

1   A paradigm, following Kuhn (1970, p. 175), is 'the entire constellation of beliefs, values, techniques, and so on shared by members of a given community'.
2   For the sake of brevity the term nursing will be used throughout this text to denote the nursing, midwifery and health visiting professions.

activism and lay knowledge acting to pursue scientific knowledge and political change.

Few nurses, even those who have completed diploma or degree courses, have had the opportunity to study either clinical or social epidemiology. Yet this subject is central to much of the work within nursing, particularly in the community but also in the hospital setting. Several approaches to healthcare research fall within the boundaries of the subject, and many nurse researchers have unwittingly utilised epidemiological designs in their work. Traditional epidemiology has retained its quantitative methodologies within a 'positivist' framework, and as such will have much to offer nurse researchers following a similar path. Those who adopt more qualitative approaches often eschew epidemiology, regarding its methods as anathema to the understanding of a social world. Likewise, many epidemiologists dismiss qualitative designs as mere anecdote. However, both approaches have their strengths and limitations, and more recently arguments for the necessity of both methodologies have been put forward (Jones and Moon, 1987).

The Briggs Report (1972) catalysed the movement to create nursing as a research-based profession. Numerous official documents since then (for example, *A Strategy for Nursing* (Department of Health, 1989a) and the *Report of the Taskforce on a Strategy for Research in Nursing, Midwifery and Health Visiting* (Department of Health, 1993a)) have reiterated the call for nursing practice to be grounded in scientific research. The mechanisms by which this may be achieved are less clear, and widely debated (Hardey and Mulhall, 1994). Should all qualified nurses undertake research? What constitutes research awareness? Who should translate research for practice and how should this be achieved? Whatever the outcome of these discussions it is clear that a considerable body of nurses, health visitors and midwives will find it increasingly important to read, understand and evaluate research articles. For the busy professional, however, keeping abreast of 'the literature' has become a daunting task. Clinical epidemiology offers a set of skills which enable healthcare workers to read and organise this material in a systematic way.

But clinical epidemiology provides more than a framework for research or a method for literature evaluation. It is a practical tool which all health workers, including nurses, can and should make use of in their everyday practice. The nursing process encompasses a cycle of assessing, planning, implementing and evaluating care (Roper *et al.*, 1990). Medicine has its own cycle of history-taking/examination, diagnosis, treatment and evaluation. Although the aims and strategies of medicine and nursing differ dramatically, and their focus on the particular or the whole respectively mark out this difference, parts of their 'processes' are remarkably similar. Both rely on gathering information of various types (for example, the results of biochemical tests, physical signs and symptoms, cultural histories, social circumstances) through an interaction with the patient, either alone or with his or her family. Such interactions may be formal, such as occurs on entry into hospital, or they may form a more subliminal part of everyday ongoing interactions with the client. The information thus elicited forms the basis for answering certain questions. In the case of medicine these might be: 'Is this person sick?'; 'Would further tests back up my "clinical" diagnosis?'; or 'What is the optimal form of therapy for this condition?'. In clinical nursing the patient has frequently already been assigned a label or diagnosis, and perhaps a treatment, by the doctor. Nevertheless, similar types of question arise concerning the nature, frequency and format of the nursing care needed to assist clients to fulfil their individual physical, psychological or social requirements. Although the frameworks of Midwifery and Health Visiting are rather different, with their emphasis on screening for and promoting 'normality' (for example, by advising on diet in pregnancy, or by monitoring the growth of babies born prematurely), the process of information gathering remains central.

This information forms the basis of the decisions that healthcare workers make, either in conjunction with their clients or in isolation. The course of action that individual nurses take varies with each new encounter, and is influenced by their own knowledge bases and experience, the experience of colleagues, the structural and processual sociocultural context of the encounter, the research literature available on the subject and many other factors. Nurses are attempting to particularise to each individual their prior experience as derived from similar encounters. Are there strategies which make this process and thereby the process of care more effective? Clinical epidemiology aims to provide a scientific basis for the subject of clinical 'observations' (defined in the broad sense discussed above). Fletcher *et al.* (1988, p. vi), discussing clinical epidemiology and medicine, state that the former is concerned with 'the best possible evidence about the actual effectiveness and efficiency of medical care and health services at a time of increasing complexity of what we might do for patients and an increasing recognition that we should not do many things and we cannot do all'. In other words, it is a method of scrutinising the validity of the clinical judgements which all healthcare professionals make in their everyday practice.

The history of traditional epidemiology and the recent development of social and lay epidemiology provide the basis for a fundamental challenge of many of the taken-for-granted precepts which underlie the current provision of healthcare in the UK, for, since its inception in 1948, the National Health Service has been concerned not with health, but with medical services. Indeed, the British Medical Association in the 1930s argued this very case. Preventative medicine and health promotion have, with some notable exceptions (for example, the vaccination programmes), taken a back seat. After the NHS was set up the vigorous and effective work of the early medical officers of health petered out or was suppressed and ignored (cf. The Black Report, 1980; The NACNE Report, 1983).

However, since the dramatic decline in the rates of infectious diseases, the challenges to improve health and prevent illness are predominantly to be found in more complex problems such as cancer and heart disease. Although it may be argued that all biological disease is only manifested as sickness through the social world (Frankenberg, 1980; Young, 1982), the contributions of both biology and sociology to an explication of the underlying causality of these more complex diseases is more readily understood.

A complication arises therefore as disciplines such as sociology and medicine, with fundamentally different epistemologies and differing theoretical approaches, attempt to tackle the same problems. The difficulties do not lie only with paradigm incompatibility; each profession will be jealously guarding its particular territory and area of expertise against intrusion from outsiders. However, it is often at the boundaries of disciplines – nursing, medicine, sociology, epidemiology – that more radical interpretations and innovative strategies are born. The relationship between disciplines such as anthropology and epidemiology remains largely neglected (Trostle, 1986). Similarly, although nursing has a patchy history of utilising epidemiological designs, there has been little or no exploration of mutual or overlapping concepts and the new insights which they might bring to both disciplines.

To summarise, nursing in its consideration of epidemiology might benefit from any or all of the following:

- a model for quantitative nursing research
- a strategy for evaluating the clinical nursing research literature
- a framework for making clinical decisions
- a mechanism for the effective and efficient planning and delivery of nursing services to **those who most need them**.
- an opportunity to enrich current nursing concepts, or to create new and mutually enhancing shared theory.

ABOUT THIS BOOK

The purpose of this book is to explore epidemiology, its knowledge base, ideology and practice in a nursing context. The book may be read in its entirety, or separate chapters may be consulted as required. However, the text does follow a logical sequence in situating epidemiology within nursing and the wider concepts of health and sickness; examining its role in the planning and delivery of healthcare in the new NHS; and finally considering a specific aspect of such care – nursing and the research associated with it. Although methods will be discussed and explained where appropriate, the overall aim is to explain epidemiology in terms of its importance and relevance to nursing in the 1990s. The approach will encompass an examination of specific issues important to both epidemiology and nursing rather than provide a 'recipe book' on how to do epidemiological studies. This latter information is readily available in many clinical or medical texts on epidemiology.

Chapter 1 introduces the subject matter of epidemiology through a consideration of its history and the essential principles, concepts and research designs which underpin the discipline. Some initial indication is also given as to the potential interactions between epidemiology and nursing. In all epidemiological studies it becomes necessary sooner or later to define whether an individual is abnormal (in traditional parlance, diseased), or normal (disease-free). However, the concepts of disease and health are widely defined and hotly debated. Chapter 2 explores these issues through a critical appraisal of the concepts of disease, illness, sickness and health as derived from a number of epistemological stances. Although portrayed as objective and value-free, epidemiology and its practice is as much socially constructed as scientifically mediated. Similarly, the professional and research strategies of nursing may be constrained by organisational boundaries. It is in this context that the evolution of nursing in the NHS and how epidemiology may add to or impede future trends in development are examined in Chapter 3.

The reorganisation of the health service has resulted in an increasing emphasis on the 'hard' data of statistics, both as a benchmark for monitoring the quality of care, and as information for planning services. Epidemiology is the 'feeder' discipline for much of this work. Chapter 4 includes a pragmatic description of the derivation and compilation of healthcare statistics, but extends the discussion to question the social and political dimensions of health information. Many of the arguments raised in Chapter 4 are continued in Chapter 5, which extrapolates on how and where epidemiology may make the maximum contribution in planning an effective health service. This leads on to a fundamental question – is rational planning possible? In an attempt to answer this, the second half of Chapter 5 explores such areas as health need, health gain and quality.

Chapter 6 turns to the more specific applications which epidemiology may have for nursing. It continues the arguments first raised in Chapter 2 concerning the different paradigms through which health and disease may be conceptualised, and attempts to situate epidemiology and nursing in this debate. Although there are many areas where epidemiology and nursing might fruitfully combine, three particular topics – health technology assessment; surveillance and control; and risk, prevention and screening – are chosen to be discussed in detail. The last chapter of the book focuses on a highly topical issue – research evaluation and utilisation. Suggesting that nursing might benefit from a more widespread appreciation and application of the methods of literature evaluation and synthesis first developed in epidemiology, the chapter also warns of the constraints of these strategies. The final section addresses the enigma of implementation through a consideration of research, knowledge and practice.

As the book developed it became clear that for each subject tackled there was a 'conventional account' which emerged from the traditional sources of epidemiological literature (i.e. journals and books either written for, or strongly influenced by, medicine), and an 'alternative account' which was gleaned from the perspectives of sociology, anthropology and occasionally nursing. This latter aspect was more difficult to unearth and appeared in widely disparate locations throughout the literature. All the chapters are presented in a particular format suited to their subject matter, but each contains elements of both the conventional and alternative accounts. On some occasions the distinctions between these two are quite clear, while on others the two accounts merge throughout the text. The two positions taken essentially rest on differing paradigms or world views – the rational science of biomedicine[3], and the naturalism/interpretism characteristic of much social science. Traditionally, nursing has had little time for epidemiology, perceiving it as both a discipline, and a practice firmly embedded in positivistic science. Nursing, however, is an eclectic discipline which has drawn on many epistemologies and methodologies in its quest for a holistic perspective. Increasingly, the sterile polemic surrounding the quantitative/qualitative debate in nursing is subsiding as flexible practitio-

---

3   The term biomedicine refers to the predominant theory and practice of medicine in Euro-American societies.

ners move the discipline forward to a more integrated approach. It is nursing, I believe, which has the potential to bring these two epidemiological discourses together, not just for the profession itself, but for those other groups working alongside nursing in the health service, and above all for the recipients of those services.

ACKNOWLEDGEMENTS

My grateful thanks are due to all of the following who kindly agreed to comment on particular aspects of the manuscript relevant to their areas of expertise:

Dr Nicky Cullum, Centre for Health Economics, University of York
Dr Helen Glenister, Anglia and Oxford Regional Health Authority, Cambridge
Mr Michael Hardey, Department of Sociology and Social Policy, University of Southampton
Dr John de Louvois, Central Public Health Laboratories, Colindale
Ms Teresa Moor, East Riding Health Authority, Hull
Ms Lynda Taylor, Central Public Health Laboratories, Colindale
Mrs Cheryl Thornton, The Nuffield Health Centre, Witney, Oxon

I am indebted to them for their time and for providing many comments which have undoubtedly improved the final version of this text.

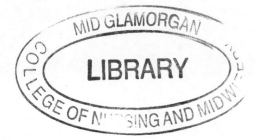

CHAPTER ONE

Introducing epidemiology

EPIDEMIOLOGY: WHAT IS IT?

Although definitions are frequently unenlightening, no text on epidemiology would be complete without its statutory 'one-liner'. Epidemiology has been defined as 'the study of the distribution and determinants of the health related states and events in defined populations, and the application of this study to the control of health problems' (Last, 1987, p. 29). It is a term derived from the Greek (*epi*=upon; *demos*=people; *logos*=science). In contrast with nursing and medicine, epidemiology is concerned with **populations** rather than individuals. Consequent on this, epidemiologists, to a greater extent than doctors and nurses, are interested in all members of a group, be they 'healthy' or 'sick'. Some of the people which they study would therefore not normally have come to the attention of the health services. Another particular difference between epidemiology and medicine is that the former often wishes to know *whether* something has occurred, rather more than the *mechanism* through which it occurred.

This emphasis on the differences between epidemiology and other healthcare disciplines belies the fact that in many areas these fields interrelate and have much to offer each other. In investigating diseases and the various lifestyles or environmental conditions associated with them, epidemiology generates information which may be used not only by public health officials but also by nurses and doctors. Healthcare planners require specific data concerning the distribution of certain conditions in order to estimate the extent and nature of the services required to meet such needs. Epidemiology provides methods for measuring disease frequency and its social and healthcare consequences. For example, epidemiological methods could be used to estimate the extent and distribution of different types of urinary incontinence in a District Health Authority. This information might be

1

used not only to determine the resources required by patients, but also in justifying the creation of posts such as a nurse continence advisor. In studying the natural course of conditions epidemiology may also identify prodromal signs and symptoms which may be applied to the early diagnosis and thus treatment of conditions. As a corollary to this, certain risk factors associated with the subsequent development of a condition may be recognised. Data of this type are invaluable in devising strategies both for the screening of potentially vulnerable groups, and for developing health promotion programmes for those at greater than average risk. For example, the recognition that ovarian cancer may develop partly as a result of a genetic disposition (Simpson and Photopulos, 1976), indicates that the screening of women whose sisters or mothers have already developed the disease might aid in earlier detection and treatment.

In these ways the basic science of epidemiology may be used in the interpretation of clinical phenomena and result in the development of more effective and efficient nursing and medical practice. As Sackett *et al.* (1991, p. x) note, 'If rational clinical practice requires the projection of diagnostic findings, prognoses and therapeutic responses from groups of patients to the individual patient, then the strategies and tactics used to understand groups of patients (that is the strategies and tactics of epidemiology and biostatistics) ought to be useful to the clinician'. Thus in the last ten years a rapidly developing field – *clinical epidemiology* – has emerged. Clinical epidemiology is 'the application of epidemiological principles and methods to problems encountered in clinical medicine' (Fletcher *et al.* 1988, p. 2). Hitherto, clinical epidemiology has stressed its importance to medicine. However, this framework may be applied equally, although perhaps with different emphasis, to nursing, midwifery and health visiting.

Another aspect of epidemiology is realised when the social and economic factors that affect health are considered. Medicine has assumed a powerful ideological and social position in today's society – some would even argue that it has taken the place of religion and law (Foucault, 1977). This hegemonic[1] discourse promulgates the idea that clinical medicine is responsible for the vast improvements in health that have occurred over the last century, and that health lies

---

1 Hegemony has been defined in various ways, but loosely it describes predominance. Thus one might speak of the biomedical hegemony imposed through Western medicine. Cultural hegemony may act quite subtly: for example, patients who consult doctors within the Western medical system do not have their views forced upon them, but already share and partake of those views.

largely within the provenance of the individual. The history of public health denies this (McKeown, 1976), and later publications such as the Black Report (1980) emphasise the strong association between socio-economic factors and health (see also Chapters 2 and 5). As Thunhurst (1991, p. 119) ominously notes 'Your birthright is still, as surely as it ever was, your death right'. *Social epidemiology*, alongside the new public health, is that branch of the discipline which considers such oft-neglected or suppressed socio-economic and cultural factors and the impact that they have on the nation's health. The following section describes how such factors formed the essential foundations to the Victorians' view of public health, and how epidemiology developed as an integral component to this project.

HISTORICAL PERSPECTIVES

Hundreds of years before the advent of the science of epidemiology people attempted to explain why disease occurred. Some cited supernatural events as the cause of sickness, while others, such as Hippocrates, attempted to delineate a rational basis, noting that disease was related to the environment and lifestyle (Adams, 1886). Although the causes of disease might have remained unknown, links between cause and effect were recognised. Based on observations of the occurrence of sickness in certain individuals and its absence in others, preventative strategies were devised. Very often religion informed these first policies in preventative health. Thus the recognition that plague had entered Europe from the Far East prompted the institution of a 30 day quarantine period on ships entering Venice from the Levant. In increasing this period to 40 days (the time Christ spent in the desert), public health practice was underpinned by religious policy and doctrine (Benenson, 1987).

The earliest phase in the epidemiological endeavour focused on infectious diseases such as cholera and typhoid. Three reasons underlie this focus: the widespread distribution of such diseases; their high mortality rate; and their propensity to occur as explosive epidemics which threaten poor and rich alike and raise a spectre of panic. The best known of these early uses of epidemiology is found in the work of John Snow. In 1854 a cholera epidemic in London allowed Snow to test his theory that this disease was disseminated via human excreta. By this time the use of quantitative methods of measuring disease frequency (rates) had been pioneered by, among others, Nightingale and Simpson. This allowed Snow to compare the incidence of cholera among the users of two water supplies. This classic epidemiological study not only defined the mechanism of transmission of the disease, but also indicated an appropriate preventative strategy (the removal of the handle from the water pump in Broad Street). In fact, the aetiological agent of cholera *Vibrio cholerae* had already been reported by an Italian named Filipo Pacini in the previous year, but the knowledge of this was not widespread, and it seems likely that Snow was unaware of it.

The exigencies of frequent epidemics of infectious disease and the requirement to control them thus linked the early development of epidemiology as a science and the concept of public health. Indeed, one of epidemiology's primary purposes, as defined by Lilienfeld and Lilienfeld (1980, p. 4), is 'to provide the basis for developing and evaluating preventative procedures and public health practices'. In the mid-19th century a public health movement based on the work of sanitary inspectors and medical officers of health gradually developed. Supported by legislation such as the National Public Health Acts of 1848 and 1875, improved disposal of sewage, supply of fresh water and cleaner streets became a priority. This Public Health Movement emphasised environmental change through largely mechanical measures, and undoubtedly had a dramatic effect upon the occurrence of epidemic infectious disease. Its ideology was not, however, one of improving the conditions under which the poor lived. Inspired by the utilitarian thinking of reformers such as Edwin Chadwick, who perceived epidemic disease as a threat to social order and capitalist production, sanitary reform was conceived as a policy for maintaining economic and moral stability.

The early history of epidemiology and public health also illustrates the crucial linkages between healthcare and socio-economic forces. Despite the facts available from Snow's epidemiological work on the transmission of cholera, the idea that disease was caused by miasmas (or bad smells and 'airs') persisted. Although this allowed the engineering aspects of sanitary reform to be successfully pursued, it essentially stifled the political or social dimensions of disease, and thereby any attempts to improve the conditions of the working classes. Indeed, as late as 1885 the British authorities were still adamant that cholera was 'non communicable, non-specific and endemic in Egypt' (the Surgeon General Sir William Hunter) (Howard-Jones, 1974). Acceptance of the epidemiological observations that cholera originated in India would have severely affected Britain's commercial interests with that country. Likewise, the idea that disease was due to atmospheric impurities fitted well with the Victorian notion that the physical conditions of the poor were the root cause of disease, rather than the particular social structures which sustained those conditions. A moral and economic dimension thus overrode certain early attempts at delineating the epidemiological processes involved in the transmission of infectious diseases.

The emphasis on environmental change and sanitary engineering within the Public Health Movement persisted until the 1870s. Subsequently, the acceptance of the germ theory of disease and the discovery of certain vaccines introduced an individualistic aspect to the prevention of ill health. This emphasis on personal preventative medicine both promoted, and was in its turn underwritten by, the ascendancy of monopoly capitalism and the associated professionalisation of medicine. Viewed from this perspective, illness was the responsibility of the individual, not a symptom of social conditions. The social aspects of epidemiological investigations were not, however, totally neglected. In the early part of the twentieth century there were several important epidemiological contributions towards an understanding of nutritional diseases, such as scurvy and pellagra. Intrinsic to such studies was an understanding that social conditions, i.e. poor nutrition, might underlie the aetiology of certain diseases. In some instances the impetus for improvements came through politico-economic necessity. Thus it was a concern with the widespread ill health of working class recruits during the Boer War that prompted the provision of school meals to improve health standards by improvements in diet (Hardy, 1981). In other cases a more philanthropic stance is in evidence, such as shown through the research of Joseph Goldberger in the US Public Health Service. Goldberger demonstrated that pellagra, until then thought to be a communicable disease to which the poor were congenitally susceptible, was due to a nutritional deficiency which was in its turn integrally related to the system of tenant farming practised in the South. Furthermore, these scientists emphasised the economic root cause of the disease '...bound up in the tenant system, which, in turn is involved in single crop agricultural production and the speculative character of agricultural finance as it is practised in the area... any measure which will improve the economic condition of the tenant farm population... will tend to lessen the prevalence of pellagra as well as ill health from most other causes' (Goldberger and Sydenstricker, 1927, p. 44).

Despite these early forays into a more social epidemiology, between 1930 and 1970 the therapeutic era of public health epitomised by hospital-based services, which focused on treatment rather than prevention, predominated. However, in the early 1970s this paradigm was increasingly challenged. McKeown's (1976) analysis of population growth and mortality concluded that immunisation and therapy had had little impact on mortality compared with the politico-economic and social factors embraced within environmental public health. This argument for the historical ineffectiveness of medicine was widened by Illich (1975), who proposed that the organisation and operation of the modern medical profession overrode the individual's control of health, and was actually responsible for a considerable amount of iatrogenic disease. Emerging from these critiques was a movement for a New Public Health which recognised that health problems were embedded not only in the physical but also in the social and psychological environments (Ashton and Seymour, 1991). This movement also found expression in the World Health Organisation's *Targets for Health for All, 2000* (WHO, 1985). This asserted that health developments were made 'not only for, but also by the people' (WHO, 1985, p. 11). A more participative and social public health thereby entered the arena. Although traditional epidemiologists were increasingly recognising the roles that social and environmental factors played in the genesis of sickness, the New Public Health catalysed ideas behind a *new social epidemiology*. Much of the momentum for this has come from social scientists. Moving beyond the consideration of static social factors as determinants of disease, the new social epidemiology seeks to understand what lies behind them. As Scott-Samuel notes (1989, p. 36), the new public health requires a new 'truly social, truly critical development in epidemiology', and this has paved the way to a new conceptualisation of epidemiology: *popular epidemiology*, which is a synthesis of political activism and lay knowledge and acts to pursue scientific knowledge and political change. Brown (1992, p. 269) defines popular epidemiology as 'the process whereby lay persons gather scientific data... and marshal the resources of experts in order to understand the epidemiology of disease'. The significance of lay knowledge is expanded on in Chapters 2 and 6, while a wider discussion of lay epidemiology will be found in Chapter 5.

The last fifty years have seen epidemiology struggling to free itself from a simplistic one agent/one disease model as it attempts to unravel chronic illnesses such as heart disease and cancer, which have no obvious single cause. Its remit has widened beyond organic disease to include mental illness and the study of such characteristics as blood group serotypes and weight which may be related to health. This new eclectic model embraces the idea that socio-economic and cultural factors may intermingle with biology in the determination of illness. Its practice thus involves participation from a wide range of healthcare professionals, including doctors, nurses, social workers, policy-makers and anthropologists among others. This multidisciplinary approach strengthens epidemiology's theoretical base, but may conceal covert aspects of its enterprise. Stallones (1980; p. 76) notes how the training and experience of physicians (who dominate the profession) render them 'deeply imprinted and reluctant to accept that most biomedical research is irrelevant to the solution of community health problems'. The dominant biomedical model also yokes epidemiology to disease classifications rooted in clinical medicine which pays scant regard to the social and economic aspects involved. The 'medical gaze' is in the West understandably focused on those particular facets of ill-health which are amenable to intervention by modern biomedicine, and it is this same gaze which has tended to dominate epidemiology.

This brief account illustrates how the history of epidemiology is not merely a linear story of logical advances to knowledge and their progressive incorporation into health policy. Political and ideological factors may both stifle new epidemiological evidence, or privilege accounts which will support the establishment of new policies. As Levine and Lilienfeld (1987; p. 2) remark: '...health policy (does not) automatically adjust to the changing base of epidemiology'. However, the same authors add that, 'If we could make use of existing epidemiological knowledge with all its limitations, the effects on society's health would be enormous'.

EPIDEMIOLOGY AND NURSING

Earlier in this chapter it was noted that epidemiology is concerned predominantly with populations rather than individuals. In contrast, nursing has placed the individual as central to its enterprise, not only in the mode by which care is delivered, as in primary nursing, but also in the philosophy of holistic care designed to meet all the physical, psychological, social, emotional and spiritual needs of its clientele. At first glance, therefore, it would appear that epidemiology would have little to offer to such an in-depth, one-on-one scenario. However, this section will illustrate how nurses, by their very position in the health-care hierarchy, and in their professional mission *vis-à-vis* patients, are in a crucial position to utilise epidemiology to its fullest extent. Statistical data are an important part of nursing's legacy and as Nightingale demonstrated provide an organised strategy for learning from experience. A significant amount of the 'routine statistics' which both nurses and doctors already collect is used by epidemiology (see Chapter 4); it is up to nurses to ensure that through a thorough understanding of the methods and principles involved they may determine that such data are put to good and proper use.

Two obstacles to the more effective recognition and use of epidemiology within nursing may have been unwittingly constructed by nurses themselves. During the last twenty years a strong movement to professionalise nursing has evolved (Beardshaw and Robinson, 1990).

Consequent on this has been the search for a particular theoretical role for nursing distinct from that of medicine. The concept of caring has been widely adopted (Watson, 1979; Leininger, 1981) and provides the basis for a number of significant nursing theories (Rogers, 1970; Orem, 1985). A model of individualised care mindful of the 'whole' patient has developed to provide a holistic framework for practice. This focus on care has succeeded in establishing nursing as a discipline distinct from the 'cure' orientation of medicine (Ellis, 1992), but it has placed epidemiology at a double disadvantage. Falling within the sphere of biomedicine, from which nursing has been seeking to distance itself, epidemiological knowledge will be accorded low status. Like many aspects of everyday life in the 20th century, epidemiology has become heavily medicalised, and is, as a consequence, of little attraction to nursing. In addition nursing's almost blind adherence to the concepts of 'care' and the 'individual' obscure any wider or more liberal interpretations which might recognise the key role that observations of groups or populations might bring. Thus another linchpin of the epidemiological project is essentially lost.

Any consideration of where epidemiology might contribute towards nursing cannot be undertaken in isolation from the momentous changes which both the profession and the National Health Service (NHS) are currently undergoing. As the training of nurses becomes absorbed into higher education, thorny questions regarding the nature and distribution of the skill mix within the profession are having to be addressed. Will the move towards an all-graduate profession result in an ever-diminishing band of highly trained individuals who direct healthcare assistants in the actual 'hands on' delivery of care to patients? This would have several implications for both the generation of epidemiological knowledge, and the initiation and conduct of research within the discipline. It might be argued that, freed from mere 'body work', qualified practitioners would be in a better position to observe and record patterns of disease or symptom occurrence which could lead to new epidemiological findings. Undoubtedly an ability to 'think epidemiologically' will increase the likelihood that appropriate observations are made, and unusual occurrences are recognised as such. In this sense graduate nurses, who are most likely to have had the opportunity to learn epidemiological concepts and principles, will be at an advantage. However, if the new educational strategies result in qualified practitioners spending less time in direct patient care then the significance of certain observations may remain unreported by a workforce untrained to view with an 'epidemiological eye'.

The history of nursing research also offers insights into the tenuous links that currently exist between nursing and epidemiology. The concern to establish the professional basis of nursing in the 1960s resulted in much of its research effort being devoted to the description and evaluation of nursing courses, with few studies into the impact of nursing on its recipients being conducted. At this time quantitative methods predominated, reflecting the dominance of the biomedical model of health. Nursing care was perceived as an emotional and subjective subject not worthy of scientific scrutiny, in much the same way as the art of medicine, although recognised by clinicians, receives little attention in serious texts (Hahn and Kleinman, 1983). Early leaders, such as Abdellah and Levine (1971) and Polit and Hungler (1983) placed a heavy emphasis on scientific methodologies, but as nursing developed in its own right as a discipline the research paradigm expanded to embrace more qualitative approaches. If less than fruitful, the quantitative/qualitative debate was certainly acrimonious, with each side defending its entrenched positions at every opportunity. As many new nursing departments developed within the faculties of human, rather than natural, sciences in higher education, the cultural environment in which nurses undergo their education has thereby contributed to a disavowal of quantitative research. Additionally, where little training in epidemiology or indeed the other biosciences and statistics has been provided it is unlikely that students will employ such approaches in their future work. As a result, a long-standing distrust of quantitative research in nursing has developed. Epidemiology, with its emphasis on populations, samples and other aspects of biostatistics, must therefore appear to many nurses as anathema to their interests in the subjective experience of individual patients in their care. Ironically, the NHS Research and Development programme (Department of Health, 1991a) may subvert much of the research in nursing into a health services research agenda. Such research, by definition, is seeking 'generalisable contributions to knowledge' (Department of Health, 1993a, p. 6) and is heavily biased towards quantitative research in general and epidemiology in particular. But how many nurses have had sufficient training in their educations to take up this task? However, in order to secure any substantial funding nurses may be forced to conceptualise problems within this particular framework. Thus the advantages and disadvantages of epidemiological approaches within nursing may be thrust rather precipitously upon us.

This introductory chapter has so far attempted to explain the basic concepts underlying epidemiology and to examine its historical development alongside the public health movement. An appreciation of the current status of nursing, and research in nursing, is followed by some indications as to why epidemiology may not have been espoused with much vigour by the profession. The remaining three sections in this chapter take a more prescriptive position by describing the fundamental principles of conventional epidemiology; the main approaches to epidemiological studies; and two of its overriding concepts (causality and natural history). This is necessary to inform the discussion in later chapters of more prosaic issues surrounding the opportunities and constraints to using epidemiology in healthcare in general, and nursing in particular. It should be noted, however, that while these concepts and principles may be applied broadly within epidemiology, they are specifically integral to the quantitative designs that have characterised much of the traditional discipline to date. Further exploration of these and other concepts more closely aligned with social and critical epidemiology will be found in Chapters 2 and 3.

SOME ESSENTIAL PRINCIPLES

This book does not attempt to provide an exhaustive guide as to how to conduct epidemiological studies. There are several texts available (Barker, 1982; Mausner and Kramer, 1985) which will help in the planning of such research, and although framed in reference to medicine the same principles will apply to nursing. It is perhaps worth commenting here, however, that the advice of an experienced researcher is worth any number of textbooks. Anyone embarking on an epidemiological project for the first time would be advised to seek out such advice, or alternatively participate in a collaborative study. Before proceeding to examine some of the issues in epidemiology in relation to nursing and the restructuring of the health service it is, however, necessary to outline the discipline's fundamental principles. Some grasp of the essential nature of epidemiology is a prerequisite for understanding the advantages and disadvantages that any union with nursing might bring. Some broad areas will be considered here, while other concepts will be explained later where they relate specifically to the context of the subject under discussion.

Many of the underlying principles of epidemiology concern its focus of study – disease in **populations**. Epidemiologists are interested in the experience of groups, the differences between groups, and whether chance might have affected these differences. Crudely stated, there are three main thrusts to the subject, which can be illustrated by the following questions:

- Who becomes sick?
- Why do certain people become sick?

and

- How effective are the possible treatments available for those who are sick?

Framed in this way epidemiology portrays itself as concerned with a disease model of health. This conceptualisation has been widely criticised by nurses and others (Engel, 1980; WHO, 1979; Frankenberg, 1980; Hahn, 1983) who propose that a wider interpretation and a more positive stance of health should be adopted (see Chapter 2). These arguments and where epidemiology fits within them are more fully discussed in Chapter 2. Putting these criticisms to one side, what is necessary here is to consider the principles important to any objective examination of groups and the events which may befall them. The most basic of these are:

- populations and sampling
- validity
- reliability
- bias

and

- chance

Populations and sampling

As noted earlier, epidemiology has at its roots the study of groups of people. It is the attempt to apply the results of information obtained from these groups to the care of individuals that is encapsulated in clinical epidemiology. A **population** is the total number or quantity (large or small) of people or things in a given location. The study of populations and how they change is termed *demography*. Demography includes the study of such characteristics as population size, density, growth and distribution. The population dynamics of a given geographical area can be studied through its birth rates, death rates and migration profile. Similarly, survival rates or life expectancy for various sections of any given population can be determined through the use of demographical techniques. Demography thus has links with statistics and geography, but because of its interests in the distribution of people and their associated morbidity and mortality it has a strong association with health sciences in general and epidemiology in particular. Although research may be conducted on a whole population (for example every graduate nurse in the UK might be contacted to determine their pattern of work since leaving university), most research uses **samples**. A sample is a subset or smaller part of a population. A random sample is one in which each member of the original population has an equal chance of being drawn. Randomly selected samples are useful, for they are more likely to represent a valid picture of the population as a whole than a sample which has not been randomly selected (i.e. they possess greater external validity – see below). Chunk or convenience samples which are not randomly selected may differ from the rest of the population through some systematic error, or simply by chance.

Validity

How closely an observed or measured state of affairs corresponds with the true state of a phenomenon is termed **validity**. In other words, validity is concerned with whether a scale, a question or an instrument measures what it is claimed to measure. **Reliability** concerns consistency: to what extent do repeated measurements of the same phenomenon fall closely together? A very simple illustration of the difference between validity and reliability is provided by Oppenheim (1984). A clock which consistently showed the time as ten minutes fast (compared with, for example, Greenwich Mean Time) would be considered reliable, but not valid. Similarly, a pressure sore susceptibility scale which consistently overrated the number of people at risk of sores could be termed reliable, but again not valid. Any set of observations may differ from the true value due to two kinds of error – bias and chance. Bias is systematic error, whereas chance is random error. Valid observations are those where bias has been minimised. Reliable observations are those where chance has been minimised. Valid inferences rely on ensuring that no distortions due to bias have been introduced through the design or conduct of a study.

Two types of validity – **internal validity** and **external validity** – are recognised. Internal validity refers to the extent to which the results obtained are a true reflection of the study population itself. Threats to internal validity are posed by any source of bias – in other words, the internal validity of any study requires the absence of systematic error or bias. External validity (or generalisability) concerns how far the results obtained in the study population hold true for other people in other situations. It stands to reason that valid generalisations should be made only from studies that have internal validity. An appreciation of validity is crucial when reading and interpreting the research literature. Any study that shows signs of questionable internal validity should not form the basis for practice. However, external validity is equally important; a study may be unimpeachable in terms of its internal validity, but be highly misleading if applied to another population. For example, the rate of infections recorded in a group of babies born prematurely, even if determined using extremely reliable and valid methods, would not be a good predictor of the rate in babies born at term, or premature babies in another location. A consideration of both bias and chance is crucial in designing rigorous epidemiological studies (and thereby to evaluating their worth), and these concepts will therefore be more fully discussed in the next sections.

Bias

Selection bias

Bias is the result of any process that causes observations to differ from true values in a systematic way – i.e. bias is systematic error. Bias may occur when selecting subjects to include in a study. Many epidemiological designs compare the experience of two groups, one of which has, for example, been exposed to a certain risk factor or intervention, whereas the other has not. Since the study is seeking to determine the effect of one particular characteristic it is important that the two groups do not differ in any other ways that might affect the outcome; in other words the groups need to be comparable in all respects except that under investigation. For instance, suppose that a district nurse believes that attendance at a day centre reduces the number of illness episodes suffered by her elderly clients. She decides to compare the health records of a group of people who attend the day centre with a group who do not. However, attendance at the day centre is governed to some extent by health status, and attendees are generally healthier (perhaps more mobile, suffering less from pain or other chronic debilitating illness) than the rest of the elderly population. By comparing these two groups the effect of attending the day centre on health status would be overemphasised.

This form of bias – **selection bias** – occurs whenever the way in which subjects are selected, or not selected, for a study distorts the estimate of effect or outcome. In studies of risk, selection bias occurs when a comparison group is chosen whose exposure to the risk factor is biased for reasons other than the one of interest. For example, a nurse might hypothesise that smoking was one risk factor in the aetiology of chronic leg ulcers. She assembles a group of patients with leg ulcers, and then attempts to seek a control group without ulcers for comparison of their smoking habits. If the control group were selected from a clinic for patients with chronic bronchitis, selection bias would occur since smoking is a cause of respiratory disease and hence the controls would overestimate the smoking habits of the population from which the cases were drawn. Consequently, the strength of the association between smoking and leg ulcers would be underestimated. Selection bias is one of three commonly occurring sources of systematic error.

Measurement bias

Measurement bias is also a possibility. Take the case of a health visitor who decides to investigate the relationship between diet and hyperactivity in children. She assembles a group of children who suffer from this disorder and then tries to match them case for case with control children who are not hyperactive. The health visitor then questions the parents of the children regarding their diet to determine whether anything that they eat might be responsible for the condition. It is quite possible that because of the media attention given to this subject, parents of children who were hyperactive might report an intake of, for example, tartrazine-containing foods more readily than parents of children without the condition. That is, the cases' recall of exposure to risk factors may differ systematically from that of the controls. The results of the study would thereby be biased towards suggesting that tartrazine-containing foods were associated with hyperactivity.

Confounding

A third source of bias is **confounding**. Confounding occurs when two factors are associated, and the effect of one is confused with the effect of the other. For example, in a study of bacteriuria it was found that females catheterised by doctors had a lower rate of infections than those who had a catheter inserted by a nurse (Crow *et al.*, 1986). However, the catheterisation of female patients was most likely to be performed by doctors in the operating theatre, and that by nurses in the ward. The prescription of antibiotics to these patients also differed (those undergoing operations being more likely to be given such drugs). It was impossible therefore to determine whether the different rates of infection were related to the location of catheterisation or the person who performed the catheterisation. The two factors were confounded.

Chance or random error

Even where bias has been eliminated, random variation may result in an estimate that may misrepresent the truth. Research designs must also attempt to minimise random error, i.e. they must strive to be reliable. A health visitor may notice what she considers to be a difference in the rate of birth defects between two different populations in her district. Two explanations are possible – the rate really is different, or by chance several children with such defects have been born in one particular population. Before coming to any conclusion it is necessary to determine whether these observations were simply a coincidence or whether some factor might be causing a higher rate of birth abnormalities in one group. In other words, it is necessary to calculate how likely such observations might be. The **probability** of random variation or chance accounting for results is estimated using statistics. Statistical tests start from the premise that any change or difference observed between, say, two groups of patients occurs by chance alone (the null hypothesis). The null hypothesis states that any difference observed is only attributable to sampling errors and not to a real effect. Using the example above, the health visitor would need to determine the probability of obtaining the difference that she observed between the two populations by chance alone. If this probability is small, the hypothesis that the results occurred by chance alone, i.e. the null hypothesis, is rejected. If it is unlikely that the results occurred by chance then the difference in the rate of birth defects between the two groups *may* be real.

Many epidemiological studies compare two groups who have perhaps undergone different exposure to a risk factor for disease, or who have or have not received treatment with a new drug. Again the question is posed: are these results due to some real effect or have they occurred by chance alone? In drawing conclusions from the data two particular errors may be made. Firstly, it may be decided that there is a difference between the two groups when in reality there is not (Type I error), or secondly it may be decided that there is no difference between the groups when in reality there is (Type II error). The likelihood of a Type I error is expressed by the p value commonly seen in the results sections of research articles. p is simply a numerical way of expressing the probability that the differences observed between the two groups could have occurred through chance alone. A **significance level** of less than 0.01 therefore indicates that only one in a hundred times would you be wrong in concluding that there was a difference when in fact there was not; in other words it is very unlikely that the differences observed were due to chance alone. In contrast the probability of a Type II error indicates the chance that a real effect may have been missed. This is particularly likely in small studies, and should always be considered when 'no significant difference' is reported. Although there have been recent improvements in the consideration of Type II errors when reporting studies, a survey by Freiman *et al.* in 1978 noted that, of 71 published drug trials reporting no benefit, 94% had a one in ten risk of missing a real therapeutic improvement of 25%.

Unlike bias, which will result in observations being more likely to be either above or below their true values, chance or random error results in an observation which is equally likely to be above or below the true value. Chance therefore is as likely to deflect an observation below the true value as above it. Bias will result in either an underestimation or an overestimation of the true value. The two sources of error, chance and bias, can be (and usually are) both present in the same situation. Consider a midwife measuring blood pressure in a pregnant woman who is prone to hypertension and toxaemia. If the sphygmomanometer which she is using is poorly calibrated she may consistently record values that are higher than the true readings this is bias (the readings are reliable i.e. consistent over time, but not valid). However, random variation will also determine that consecutive readings will fluctuate around (both above and below) a mean reading – this is chance.

Valid and reliable studies

Known bias may be prevented by rigorous study design, which eliminates selection or measurement bias, and proper data analysis, which can correct for errors caused by confounding. Research articles should provide sufficient information to evaluate potential sources of bias, but naturally it is important that the reader is sufficiently skilled to recognise the importance of this effect and how, and where to look for it. However, as Fletcher *et al.* (1988, p. 12) note, 'no amount of statistical analysis can correct for unknown biases in data'. They intimate that statistics should not be applied to data from studies that are poorly designed since this may promote a 'false respectability to misleading work'.

Chance is inherent in making observations on a 'sample of reality', but it can be reduced to an acceptable level by proper design. A statistically reliable study aims to maximise the precision of the results through minimising random error, but there is always the finite possibility of error, and it is statistics which allows this error to be estimated. A major error in epidemiological designs concerns sampling, and the existence of this sampling error indicates that attention needs to be paid to ensuring that Type I and Type II errors fall within acceptable limits. These issues are considered further in the next section. As a final note, the warning above concerning validity needs reiterating. Statistical precision (and, related to this, reliability) is obviously an issue, but readers should be aware that it is perfectly possible to get a very precise estimate of the wrong answer! The validity of any study is therefore of overriding importance, and epidemiologists spend much time and effort in their attempts to eliminate systematic error to ensure validity.

Experienced researchers make use of their knowledge of bias and chance to recognise and correct for much of the error that may enter epidemiological studies through poor design or faulty analysis. In the same way, readers of such research must critique and evaluate studies according to similar criteria. Chapter 7 will explore how this may be done in more detail.

THE MAJOR APPROACHES TO EPIDEMIOLOGICAL STUDIES

As discussed above, it is not the purpose of this text to provide detailed information concerning how epidemiological studies should be designed and conducted. There are numerous books (e.g. Barker, 1982; Morton and Hebel, 1984; Mausner and Kramer, 1985; Hulley and Cummings 1989) which contain such information, even if they are focused on medical rather than nursing issues. A more recent text from the USA (Harkness, 1995) does locate epidemiological designs within nursing. Although the specific details of epidemiological designs will not be discussed here, the format of the main types of study and the kind of research questions which they might be expected to answer will be outlined.

Two main types of epidemiological research are recognised – **observational studies** and **experimental studies**. This section will briefly examine the different types of design that fall under these two broad headings. Further discussion, with specific examples of where nursing might use these particular approaches, will be found in Chapter 6. The experimental approach has been used widely in epidemiology, and some nurse researchers have also undertaken experimental studies (Sleep *et al.*, 1984; Flint *et al.*, 1989; Harding *et al.*, 1989). However, human populations cannot always be easily studied through experiments. Very often, logistical and ethical obstacles prevent the researcher from achieving the control necessary to this design. Epidemiologists have therefore developed rigorous observational approaches to control, or at least recognise the many sources of bias that may invalidate the study of natural events through the 'scientific method'.

Observational studies

Observational studies involve the gathering of data *au naturel*, i.e. events are simply observed as they happen, and the researcher plays no active role in what takes place. Who is (or who is not) exposed to, for example, a factor which might put them at increased risk of developing a certain condition is not manipulated by the investigators, but left to life's course. As a result of this, observational studies are more liable to bias than are experiments. In the natural course of events those people exposed to a risk factor might differ from unexposed people in a variety of ways. When comparing the two groups it would then be impossible to determine which particular difference was related to the development of the condition. For example, it might be recorded that one group of elderly patients with intransigent leg ulcers had a lower nutritional status than another group who did not suffer this condition. However, it would be important to establish whether differences in any other factors between the two groups, such as poor circulation or immobility, might have been responsible for the effect observed. Three main approaches to observational studies have been adopted by epidemiologists: **cohort studies**, **case control studies** and **prevalence studies**. In each case, attempts must be made to recognise, and deal with, the potential differences between comparison groups that might arise. Both cohort studies and case control studies may be used to determine risk factors, i.e. factors that are associated with an increased risk of developing a certain condition or disease.

Cohort studies

A cohort is a defined group of people who have something in common (for example five-year-olds entering education for the first time or women in the third stage of labour). The characteristics which the members of the group have in common may take many different forms, including age, presence of a particular disease, geographical area of residence and dietary habits. In a cohort study, subjects without the outcome of interest are assembled, classified according to characteristics which might be related to outcome, and then observed through time to determine which of them experience the outcome of interest. Such studies may be prospective – the cohort is assembled in the present and followed into the future (a concurrent cohort study), or retrospective – the cohort is assembled from past records and followed forward from that time (an historical cohort study). Figure 1.1 illustrates these two designs. What characterises cohort studies is that subjects are categorised on the basis of the independent variable[2]. For example, patients in a study of the development of pressure sores (Cullum and Clark, 1992) were categorised according to various factors, such as blood pressure, weight, serum protein concentration

---

2   Studies which examine the relationship between variables in any given situation often invoke the speculation that a cause and effect relationship may exist. The causative variable is usually termed the **independent variable** and the outcome is termed the **dependent variable**.

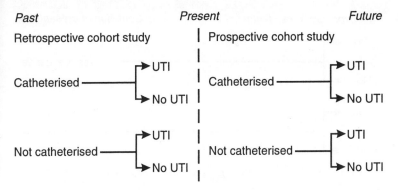

Figure 1.1 *Schematic diagram of a prospective and retrospective cohort study concerning urethral catheterisation as a risk factor for urinary tract infection (UTI).*

and use of special support mattresses, and then observed for the occurrence of pressure sores.

Two of the disadvantages of cohort studies include the length of time that may be necessary to conduct the study and the subsequent costs that will accrue, and the necessity for large-scale studies when the outcome of interest occurs infrequently (for example the Framingham heart study (Dawber, 1980) followed 5000 adults over many years). Although cohort studies are subject to bias this is a much greater problem in case control studies (see below).

Case control studies

In case control studies a group of people with the particular condition of interest are assembled (the cases) and compared with an otherwise similar group without the condition (the controls). Figure 1.2 illustrates a case control study.

In contrast to a cohort study, the case control design categorises subjects according to the dependent variable, and factors in the past (independent variables) which may explain the outcome are sought. Case control studies are therefore always retrospective. The time frame for case control studies and cohort studies is outlined in Table 1.1.

Case control studies have a number of advantages which all relate to the fact that the design centres on the identification of *cases at the present time*. It is logistically simpler and economically cheaper to assemble cases and then seek controls, than it is (as in the cohort design) to observe a much larger group of unaffected individuals and

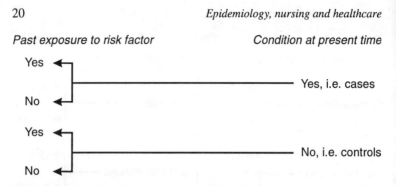

Figure 1.2 *Schematic outline for the design of a case control study.*

Table 1.1 *Time frame for cohort and case control studies*

Type of study	Past	Present	Future
Cohort		Identify the exposure of study subjects to risk factor	Measure outcome
Case control	Collect information on past exposure	Select subjects according to presence (case) or absence (control) of condition	

wait for cases to occur. In other words, the natural frequency of disease (which may be very low) does not constrain the identification of cases. In addition, the latency of the outcome will not affect case control studies – the cases are assembled at the start. Cohort studies in comparison might need to be conducted over a long period of time while the outcome of interest is awaited. For example, the time lag between the exposure to risk factors, such as carcinogens, and the development of disease may be many years.

However, case control studies are particularly prone to biases. Since the 'case' and 'control' group are chosen by the investigator, there is considerable scope for selection bias to occur. It is important that both the cases and the controls have had an equal chance of being exposed to the factor of interest. A particular problem is selective survival, whereby those who survive long enough to be selected into the sample represent a distorted (either under- or over-) representation of exposure to the risk factor. Even if selection bias is avoided, problems may occur in assuring the validity of measuring exposure after the outcome has occurred (measurement bias). Measurement bias which may occur as a result of cases recalling exposure differently from non cases was discussed above. Not surprisingly sick people have generally reflected more on events and occurrences either medical e.g. drug histories, or non medical e.g. working conditions, than controls who are not sick. A second source of measurement bias in case control studies concerns how the presence of the outcome may influence recording of the exposure. Interviewers aware of a putative relationship between risk factors and a particular outcome may pursue this line of enquiry more assiduously and carefully than if they were in ignorance of the patient's outcome status. As far as possible, therefore, data collectors should be kept in ignorance of the exposure status of the individual and/or blinded to the specific hypothesis under investigation.

Prevalence studies

A third type of observational design is the cross-sectional or **prevalence study**. Such studies are common in both medical and nursing research. Fletcher *et al.* (1988) report that this particular design accounts for almost one third of the research articles in major medical journals.

In prevalence studies a defined population is surveyed and their exposure or 'disease' status is determined at one point in time. Subjects both with and without the condition of interest are included in the survey giving a 'snapshot' of a certain moment in time. A prevalence is the proportion of the population that has a condition at a certain point in time (point prevalence). In contrast, incidence is the fraction of a group free of a condition that develops it over a given period of time (a day, a year, a decade). By definition, therefore, an incidence survey is longitudinal, rather than cross-sectional. Incidence measures the rate at which new cases arise in a population, as opposed to prevalence, which measures the proportion of a population which has the condition at any one point in time. Prevalence studies are mainly useful in planning healthcare services and informing policy issues (see Chapters 4 and 5).

However, only those cases alive and uncured at the time of the survey will be recognised. They may also be used to investigate relationships between risk factors and outcomes, but in this case two biases may be particularly troublesome. Since outcome and the factors responsible for it are measured at the same time, it may be difficult to work out the temporal sequence of these two events. Which came first – the disease or the risk factor? (See the following section for a discussion of causality and temporality.) In addition, the cases noted in a prevalence survey may be a biased subset of the whole population, since prevalence is affected by the duration of the condition; in other words the factors associated with prevalence may be the same factors associated with survival. In general, prevalence surveys tend to under-estimate acute diseases, such as fatal coronary events, but diseases of long duration, such as arthritis, would be better represented. Incidence surveys, in contrast, because of their longitudinal design, are able to illuminate the time course of events and to distinguish between old and new cases of disease.

Experimental studies

Unlike observational studies, in experimental studies researchers do have control over who is and who is not exposed to the factor under investigation. Two types of experimental study are common in epidemiology – clinical trials and preventative trials.

Clinical trials study the effect of a specific treatment intervention on people who already have a particular condition. Traditionally, such trials tested the efficacy and safety of drugs, but increasingly other 'treatments', such as equipment, or 'procedures', such as strategies for delivering care, have been examined using clinical trials. For example, the blockage of urinary catheters with inorganic deposits is a distressing problem which frequently affects patients being cared for at home (Getliffe, 1992). A recent trial (Bull *et al.*, 1991) compared two types of urinary catheter to determine how long they remained *in situ*, and the extent to which they became encrusted. Their results suggested that newer hydrogel catheters remained *in situ* longer than silicone elastomer-coated catheters. Trials of procedures are particularly difficult to conduct rigorously. However, the study by Bond *et al.*, (1989a; 1989b), comparing the care received by frail elderly people in long stay wards of general hospitals with that in three experimental NHS nursing homes, illustrates that such trials are feasible and can yield useful results.

Preventative trials investigate the effect of a potential preventative measure on people who do not have, as yet, the condition in question. For example, a trial might be set up to examine the effect of two different types of pressure-relieving mattresses on the subsequent incidence of pressure sores in elderly patients.

Both clinical and preventative trials are experiments that are conducted in the real world rather than in the laboratory. The experimental approach, first expounded by Campbell and Stanley (1963), is regarded by many quantitative researchers as the optimum research design, since it provides the framework through which cause and effect relationships may be tested. It achieves this through verifying in very precise terms the relationship between variables (dependent and independent) in any given situation. The investigator has control over the independent variable (perhaps a new drug treatment), which is manipulated to determine its effect on the dependent variable (the outcome for the patient). To ensure rigour, the impact of the independent variable must be measured through valid and reliable techniques. In addition, the effects that any factors other than the independent variable might be exerting must be minimised. To achieve these stringent criteria two essential features must be realised – randomisation and control.

Randomisation is necessary in the effort to produce an experimental group and a control group that have similar characteristics. Where randomisation is successful, a study will possess internal validity (that is, it is relatively certain that the results of the study were due to the effect of the independent variable).

Control is exerted by the researcher over the environment, the independent variable and internal validity (Cook and Campbell, 1979). The pay-off for this control is the ability to test hypothesised relationships in a rigorous manner.

Clinical and preventative trials that achieve successful randomisation and control encapsulate all the features of the experimental approach, and thus the data they generate have high reliability. The randomised controlled trial (RCT) is therefore considered by many to be the optimum strategy for testing hypotheses in the clinical arena. It has been widely used by medical epidemiologists to evaluate new or old drugs, but it is a technique that is relatively neglected by nurses.

The conduct of trials includes the selection of subjects, their separation into compatible groups, the application of the intervention to the experimental group and the measurement of outcome in both groups. Except for the intervention, the prime objective is to treat the control, or comparison, group in the same way as the experimental group. Figure 1.3 illustrates a randomised control trial to determine the effect of pre-operative washing with antibacterial soap on subsequent wound sepsis rates.

Swartz *et al.* (1980) have described two approaches to clinical trials – pragmatic and explanatory. For various reasons, not everyone assigned to a specific 'treatment' group will receive that 'treatment'. Explanatory trials involve the comparison of two clearly defined treatments from a theoretical standpoint. In this case the analysis compares those who received the intervention with those who did not (regardless of which group they were randomly allocated to). The question being asked is 'did those who actually received the treatment

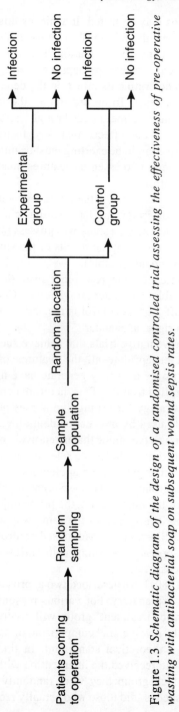

Figure 1.3 *Schematic diagram of the design of a randomised controlled trial assessing the effectiveness of pre-operative washing with antibacterial soap on subsequent wound sepsis rates.*

do better?'. The problem is that the trial is no longer randomised, and has in a sense reverted to a cohort study. Explanatory trials must therefore guard against the biases that afflict this particular non-experimental design.

In pragmatic trials the comparison is made under conditions which might normally prevail in practice and the groups as originally conceived by the protocol are compared (for example, see Bond *et al.*, 1989a,b). This has the advantage of mimicking more closely what happens in real life, and also that the trial remains 'randomised'.

Although the criteria discussed above for the experimental approach apply equally to RCTs, conducting an experiment in the 'social world' is trickier than manipulating inanimate objects in a laboratory. Some of the difficulties that may arise and the strategies for overcoming them are discussed below. A fuller explanation of the fundamentals (Friedman *et al.*, 1983; Fletcher *et al.* 1988), or statistical concepts (Simon, 1991) underlying randomised controlled trials may be found elsewhere. As with observational studies, the selection of subjects to include in clinical trials may be biased, thereby endangering the generalisability, or external validity of the trial. This deficiency is frequently overlooked by the novice reviewer of the literature because its presence is hidden in polished research reports. Subjects may be excluded from trials if they fail to meet specific exclusion/inclusion criteria; refuse to participate; or appear that they might not comply with the treatment. Very often entry to a trial will be restricted intentionally to increase homogeneity and thus internal validity, but this only occurs at the expense of generalisability. Those subjects who are judged to be eventual non-compliers, or who decline to participate, are likely to be systematically different from the remainder of the population. Their exclusion will further bias the sample and reduce its external validity.

The rationale behind the random allocation of subjects to experimental or control groups is to achieve comparable groups (for example with regard to age, sex, disease severity or social class). Any difference in outcome may then be attributed to the intervention alone. However, dissimilarities may arise, and a table of characteristics of treated and control groups should always be provided to check this. Sometimes these differences can be accommodated into the analysis, or alternatively, stratified randomisation may be integrated into the original design. Where it is believed that certain characteristics are strongly related to outcome patients may be grouped into strata according to these, and then randomly allocated to receive the intervention or not. This ensures that characteristics that might affect outcome do not by bad luck appear unevenly in treated and control groups.

In all trials it is important to standardise the intervention and attempt to ensure that both the investigator and the patient are unaware (blind) of which group (experimental or control) they belong to. Although clinical trials of drugs do present many problems in this regard (Friedman *et al.*, 1983), more complex interventions present formidable challenges. Bond *et al.* (1989a,b) discuss how it was relatively simple to document the structure, and to some extent the management, of the nursing homes and hospital wards in their study. However, capturing the 'process of care' and the implicit or unacknow-ledged facets of this (such as staff–patient interactions or the role of rituals) was more complicated. In this case a multidisciplinary team of researchers with experience in nursing, medicine, statistics, economics, anthropology and computing was required to design a successful strategy.

Classically, the outcome of clinical trials is discussed through the concept of the primary response variable (Friedman *et al.*, 1983). This should define and answer the primary question posed by the trial. Clear-cut end-points, such as death, resolution of a specific infection or complete closure of a wound, are most desirable because they reduce the likelihood of bias occurring during the assessment of outcome – in other words some outcomes are easier to document accurately than others. For example, Colgan *et al.* (1990), in their study of the treatment of leg ulcers with oxpentifylline, chose a clear end-point of time to complete healing. If a certain stage of healing had been chosen as the end-point, different assessors might have interpreted the stage in different ways. However, in nursing such well-defined outcomes are often not available, and are frequently irrelevant. Newell (1992) provides a useful discussion of criteria used to evaluate outcomes in healthcare research. Chapter 6 will also expand on the subject of outcome measures.

Ethical considerations

Before leaving the subject of experimental studies, it is important to raise the issue of ethics. Ethical considerations are paramount in any research study, but the nature of experimental research, which in theory divests the investigator with a degree of control over the participants, merits particular care. For some, the very nature of experimental research, in which the investigator is in a position of control over the 'subjects', is unacceptable. Naturalistic, and in particular feminist, researchers would contend that this type of research perpetuates a discourse wherein male middle class researchers are seen to dominate their largely powerless subjects. For naturalists the optimum research designs emphasise mutual participation and control, so that research is done *with* someone, not *on* them.

Where the experimental approach is adopted, particular care must be taken to ensure that participants are fully informed of the implications of joining a trial. The research must not deprive control subjects of the necessary care, i.e. it would be unethical to mount a trial if there was already good evidence that one of the treatments was superior. Participants also must be assured of their right to withdraw at any time.

The crux of the dilemma probably rests on the extent to which true 'informed consent' can be achieved when trials are conducted by healthcare professionals to whom society has designated powerful positions in relation to their clients. Despite internationally agreed regulations concerning informed consent, the validity of this concept still probably rests on the ability and commitment of the investigators to communicate honestly with participants and provide them with all the information at their disposal.

To summarise, clinical and preventative trials are central to the evaluation of drugs and certain clinical procedures. They provide valid and reliable data on which to base practice, but are time-consuming, expensive and difficult to organise. These difficulties in designing and managing trials should not, however, preclude the use of experimental research in nursing, and some examples of where this approach may be particularly appropriate will be discussed in Chapter 6.

IMPORTANT CONCEPTS IN EPIDEMIOLOGY

Causality

A prime aim of epidemiology is to study the aetiology of disease, or in other words to attempt to assign a cause to a given outcome (in this case disease). Much epidemiological research is therefore directed towards elucidating cause and effect relationships. Two types of causal relationship are recognised: direct and indirect. Direct causal associations occur where a certain factor is a direct cause of a certain disease. This is most easily illustrated in the case of infectious diseases. It was the German doctor Robert Koch who in 1882 first articulated a set of postulates for determining whether an infectious agent was the cause of a disease. He set forth four conditions which needed to be met:

1. The organism must be present in every case of disease.
2. The organism must be isolated and grown in pure culture.
3. The organism, once inoculated into a susceptible animal, must cause the disease in question.
4. The organism must then be isolated and identified from the animal.

Over the succeeding years the aetiology of many infectious diseases was clarified using these propositions. It should be noted, however, that apparent directness depends on the current state of knowledge in any particular subject. Initial investigations into outbreaks of legionnaires' disease in the early 1970s (Fraser *et al.*, 1977) suggested that its cause might lie with the water supplies in large buildings. It was not until later, when techniques to culture the bacterium *Legionella pneumophila* were developed, that the direct cause of the disease was clarified (Brenner *et al.*, 1978).

To some extent, many diseases, even those of infectious origin, may have several of these inbuilt stages in their development – in other words, the proximity of cause and effect may vary. In certain cases, host susceptibility and environmental factors may determine the subsequent outcome of events. For example, although most people eating a trifle contaminated with staphylococcal toxins will suffer ill effects, the development of a disease such as tuberculosis is not solely dependent on exposure to the tubercle bacillus. In this latter case, environmental conditions, such as poor housing and nutrition, are important components in the concept of causality.

The above examples illustrate some of the areas where early epidemiologists had considerable success in controlling outbreaks of disease. With the advent of chronic diseases as the major cause of mortality and morbidity (in the Western world at least), the concept of a single causative factor has had to be revised. Most chronic diseases have multiple causes, and likewise particular causative factors may cause more than one disease. Coronary heart disease has been related to several causes – smoking, obesity, high blood pressure and stress, to name just some. But similarly smoking not only causes heart disease but also bladder cancer, lung cancer and chronic respiratory complaints. Multiple causes may interact in more than a simply additive way – the risk may be potentiated beyond that which would be expected if more than one risk factor is present. MacMahon and Pugh (1970) have described this interrelationship between many causative factors, some known and some unknown, and the disease outcome as the 'web of causation'.

Establishing a cause and effect relationship in clinical practice, where many different variables may be existing in a single situation and where ethical, structural or financial constraints may be present, is much less easy than in laboratory work, where considerable control may be exerted. The limiting factor in determining the evidence for causal relationships is the strength of the research design adopted for the study. Randomised controlled trials, which are in effect clinical experiments, provide the most powerful way of establishing causal relationships. Designs that are not experimental exhibit more or less propensity for potential biases to enter the data, thus weakening the evidence for a cause and effect relationship. However, because epidemiologists frequently have to investigate situations where the experimental approach is either unethical or unfeasible they have developed rigorous observational designs. Unlike experiments or randomised controlled trials where the independent variable is under the control of the investigator, in observational studies the subject is exposed to the independent variable through, perhaps, geographical location, genetic endowment or occupational exposure. Control subjects must then be sought who are similar in every respect to the exposed subjects except in the factor of interest.

For example, a midwife might hypothesise that babies born to mothers who had premature rupture of membranes might suffer more complications than babies born to mothers who remained intact until term. It would not be ethical to artificially rupture the membranes of one group of mothers in order to set up a true experiment. Instead, the midwife would have to study a cohort (a defined group of people) of mothers over time. Some of these women would suffer premature rupture of membranes (i.e. the risk factor was present), while others would not. The outcome of interest, i.e. postnatal complications for the baby, could then be recorded in each group.

Cohort studies provide the next best evidence to experiments because the effects of bias (selection, measurement and confounding) can be minimised in their design. Other epidemiological designs, such as case control and cross-sectional studies, are more subject to bias and, as a result, provide weaker evidence for cause and effect relationships. Cohort studies are probably the most widely used epidemiological design in nursing research (Jacobsen and Meininger, 1985).

Since much of epidemiological research rests on observational rather than experimental studies, guidelines have been developed to assess the evidence for or against cause. These criteria were developed by Sir Austin Bradford, an English statistician, in 1965 (Hill, 1965). Before proceeding further, however, it is perhaps worth restating the relationship between association and cause.

In the investigation of cause and effect relationships, epidemiologists use statistics. Initially they are interested to know whether any relationship exists between two factors. An example of this process can be seen in the investigation of an apparently increased rate of urethral strictures observed in men undergoing open heart surgery in the early 1980s (Edwards *et al.*, 1983; Blacklock, 1986). Was open heart surgery a cause of these strictures? Statistical tests are used to determine whether any recorded relationship between two such factors occurred with a frequency greater than would be expected by chance alone. However, even if the two factors are associated statistically (as they were in this case), they may not be associated causally. The second step is to ensure that selection and measurement biases have not given rise to an apparent association which in reality does not exist. Finally, it must be determined that the suspected causal factor is not related indirectly to the outcome (or effect) through another (confounding) factor. In the example above, for instance, the urethral strictures were not caused by the type of operation that the subjects were undergoing, but by the use of a certain type of urethral catheter in such patients which leached chemicals into the urethra, causing the strictures to occur (Talja *et al.*, 1985).

Keeping in mind this information regarding association and cause, let us return to how epidemiological evidence may be scrutinised for causal inferences. Bradford suggested eight criteria for determining whether a factor is the cause of a disease. These may be used to examine and synthesise the findings of several studies on the same topic, thereby strengthening or diminishing the case for causality. It should be noted that the criteria do not all carry equal weight.

Temporality

It would seem fundamental that any cause should precede its hypothesised effect. For instance, if an association is noted between the consumption of cows' milk and hypersensitivity in babies, one would not consider cows' milk as a risk factor unless its consumption had preceded the episodes of allergy observed. In many cases this principle therefore appears self-evident. However, in chronic diseases, which may have developed slowly over time, it is not always easy to determine when the precipitating event for the disease first occurred, and therefore whether any risk factor preceded this event. Fletcher *et al.* (1988) provide the example of endometrial cancer and the suggestion that it is linked with oestrogen therapy. Oestrogen therapy may be used in the treatment of uterine bleeding, but some investigators have argued that if this bleeding is caused by endometrial cancer, which is diagnosed after the commencement of oestrogen therapy, then it might be hypothesised that oestrogens caused the disease, when they did not. (Further studies have shown that this latter possibility is in fact probably not correct.) Temporal ambiguity is a particular problem in cross-sectional studies, where causes and effects are measured at the same point in time.

The strength of the association

The evidence for a causal relationship increases as the strength of the association between the two factors increases. The magnitude of this effect is measured by the relative risk ratio (i.e. how many times more likely are people exposed to the risk likely to develop disease compared with those who are not exposed?). The larger this ratio the greater the likelihood that the relationship is causal. Probability does not indicate the strength of an association; a weak relationship may be statistically significant if a large sample size has been used in the study.

The dose–response effect

Continuing the argument above, if an increasing incidence of disease is related to an increasing level of exposure to the risk factor, then the argument for a cause and effect relationship is also increased. However, an alternative explanation may exist, since a dose–response effect cannot rule out confounding factors. The absence of a dose–response effect does not exclude the possibility of cause, since the relationship may be in the form of a threshold effect.

Reversibility

If the removal of a risk factor (for example the handle of the Broad Street pump) results in a decreased incidence of disease, then it is likely that it was the cause of the disease.

Consistency

The replication of studies which come to the same conclusion, particularly if they are conducted in different settings and with different patients, is strong evidence that the relationship is causal. However, consistent results might indicate that several studies were simply biased in the same direction. Lack of consistency does not necessarily invalidate results, and in these cases it is important to scrutinise the rigour with which the study was conducted (see Chapter 7).

Coherence

The cause and effect relationship is strengthened if it is consistent with other known facts, particularly if there are other examples analogous to the one in question. For example, it is well established that urethral catheters increase the incidence of urinary tract infection; thus it is easier to suggest that other invasive devices, such as intravenous cannulae, may similarly cause infections in the bloodstream.

Biological plausibility

Here the case for cause and effect is strengthened where it is consistent with known mechanisms that might be acting. Note, however, that this premise is dependent on the current state of knowledge, which history has shown can change quite dramatically over time.

Specificity

This criterion implies that one cause has one effect. As we have discussed above, this is rarely the case and therefore lack of specificity in a proposed cause and effect relationship is not justification for rejecting it. Most health outcomes have multiple causes.

All the above criteria may be used for reviewing and evaluating the evidence for causality. Obviously, each particular issue needs to be examined logically and sensibly within the limits of its own parameters. It is not simply a matter of using the criteria as a checklist. (The following references provide further information: Lilienfeld and Lilienfeld, 1980; Mathews and Haynes, 1986; Fletcher *et al.*, 1988.)

The natural history of disease

The second important concept essential to the principles and methods of epidemiology, and therefore to a clear understanding of the subject, is the natural history of disease. This is the process whereby diseases occur and progress.

The natural history of any disease is generally defined as the way in which the condition develops without any medical intervention (Fletcher *et al.*, 1988). This distinguishes it from the clinical course of a disease, which has been defined as its evolution under medical treatment. These distinctions are, however, rather misleading, since many people other than doctors treat sickness. Treatment may be forthcoming from other professional healthcare workers, such as nurses, physiotherapists and dieticians. In addition, much healthcare is meted out by practitioners outside the mainstream of Western medicine, for example by faith healers, herbalists and homoeopaths. Not only professionals are involved, however: a major component of healthcare advice and treatment is provided by lay people – mothers, aunties, workmates.

How can we define what the *natural course* is for any particular case? Even where professional help has been sought accounts of the course of a disease may be misleading. For instance, those seeking help may be more severely affected. Samples of this type are selected, therefore, and may not represent others who have the same disease but have not yet visited their doctor. Particular problems also arise where the course of a disease is based on observations made by specialist centres, who probably see a biased sample of all people with the condition.

In order to ascertain an accurate picture of the natural course of a disease it is essential therefore to include in the sample a range of patients from widely different settings. Those attending specialist clinics, who perhaps have a more severe manifestation of disease or a particular complication, must be included with others who remain in the community and are cared for by general practitioners. Others will never come to the attention of the conventional health service, either because their disease is accepted as part of life's ordinary discomforts, or because they consult non-allopathic practitioners. For many chronic diseases, therefore, it is unlikely that a completely reliable account of their evolution can be described.

These are important considerations, for the natural course of a disease is used in **prognosis**. Prognosis is the forecasting of future events, or the prediction of the course which a disease will follow. Most patients when presented with a diagnosis, apart from trying to make sense of why they have become sick ('Why me?' 'Why now?'), will wish to know what the future holds. Will the disease become worse and how quickly? Will it kill me? Will I have good spells and bad spells, or can it go away altogether? Will I be able to carry on working? A major component of the information that both doctors and nurses provide to patients concerns the answers (or lack of answers) to such questions. Epidemiology can assist in attempting to provide the most accurate answers – to be as clear as possible that certain events may occur, or to indicate where so little information is known that other events cannot be predicted.

Personal clinical experience may provide the practitioner with the knowledge to answer some of the questions above. However, the caveats about the biased selection of patients that may present in any particular setting must be borne in mind.

Prognosis may be expressed as a rate (e.g. the case fatality rate=the number of patients with disease who die of it). It would also be useful to know, however, the probability of patients developing a certain outcome at any point in time. The simplest epidemiological method of determining such survival (and this does not simply refer to death) is to follow a cohort of patients with the condition through time and record what happens. However, this would be an extremely long task, and problems such as the drop out of patients could mean that much valuable data would have to be eventually discarded. These problems can be overcome by the use of **survival** or **life table analyses**. These estimate the onset of any event by accumulating the rates for *all* patients at risk during the foregoing time intervals.

Two further important points need to be made before closing this section. Firstly, remembering the natural history of disease, it is crucial that prognostic studies are particularly clear about the stage of disease development at which observations begin. If observations are commenced at different times in different patients, e.g. at diagnosis, at hospitalisation or at time of first symptoms, it would be extremely difficult to interpret the timing of subsequent events and thus to ascertain an accurate prognosis. Secondly, much of the biomedical literature contains information concerning outcomes which, while useful in understanding the mechanisms of the disease, is of scant use to patients. Biological phenomena are only of interest clinically where they may be directly related to symptoms perceived by patients. Only 3% of a survey of research articles in the medical literature reported outcomes related to social or occupational function (Fletcher and Fletcher, 1979).

Although a knowledge of the natural course of a disease is primarily important in prognosis, it also has implications for the diagnosis/ screening and treatment of disease. The interpretation of diagnostic tests and signs naturally depends on a prior conception of when such signs appear in the course of a disease. Without this information it would be impossible to determine in the case of a negative test whether it was truly negative or whether it was simply too early in the course of the disease to detect the effect. For example, the antibodies to the HIV virus may not appear for up to six months after exposure to the micro-organism (Bor *et al.*, 1991). If suspected cases were screened only one month after exposure, subsequent development of antibodies might be missed.

Similarly, different treatment modalities may be appropriate at different points in the natural history of a condition. This is particularly relevant in the case of cancer, where the prediction of the expected course may enable the selection of appropriate treatments at appropriate stages.

CHAPTER TWO

Issues in health and disease

Chapter 1 introduced the subject of epidemiology by tracing its history and subsequent development as an integral component of the early public health movement. A brief exploration of the potential relationship between epidemiology and nursing followed. Some of the principles and concepts important to the discipline were then examined along with a description of the research designs that are most commonly used by its practitioners. This initial description of the essentials of epidemiology will be expanded in Chapter 2 through an exploration of the fundamental constructs that underpin much of the subject. This will be achieved through a critical appraisal of the concepts of disease, illness and sickness, and their counterpart: health.

The nature of much of this material is such that a more controversial picture will emerge, which may challenge some of the conventional thinking embedded within the traditional epidemiology described in Chapter 1. Lilienfeld and Lilienfeld (1980, p. 4) define epidemiology as 'the study of a disease or a physiological condition in human populations and of the factors which influence that distribution... it can be regarded as a sequence of reasoning concerned with biological inferences derived from observations of disease occurrence and related phenomena in human population groups'. Epidemiology has often been described as the basic science of public health, and, since it is the science of health in human populations, as a social science (Tuomilehto and Puska, 1987). Undoubtedly, epidemiologists. like medical sociologists, avow the multicausal nature of the origins of disease. In addition, as Chapter 1 illustrated, the theory and practice of epidemiology has always been deeply influenced by the sociocultural and political environment in which it is conceived.

Health and ill health are central concepts around which knowledge within a number of disciplines, including medical sociology, medical anthropology, medical geography and epidemiology, is organised.

However, although these disciplines may all focus on the same fields of enquiry, their modes of reasoning and epistemologies differ. Although epidemiology does not carry a 'medical' label, like the other disciplines mentioned, its essential character is derived from biomedicine, unlike, for example, medical anthropology, which is rooted in the parent discipline – anthropology. This lack of a visible medical tag is interesting and attests to the implication that epidemiology's medical parentage is assumed in tacit knowledge of the subject. There is no need to specifically designate it with a medical label. Like Western medicine, orthodox epidemiology is firmly based on positivist principles, and its definitions, concepts and methods of inquiry reflect this.

However, recent calls for a 'critical epidemiology' have been expressed (Davies, 1982). This chapter will focus on how the central concepts of disease, illness, sickness and health are invoked through epidemiology and how the perception of these differs across the other disciplines which contribute towards theory in this area. In particular the convergence and divergence between the position of nursing and epidemiology regarding these concepts will be compared. By examining the issues surrounding health and disease, the character and assumptions upon which the various perceptions of these concepts are based will be exposed.

PERCEPTIONS OF HEALTH AND ILL HEALTH

From the various definitions already quoted, it is clear that epidemiology has a major concern with studying those who do and do not become diseased, and the possible reasons for or causes of (social, environmental, physical) why this occurs. Epidemiology is thus oriented to disease, itself a biomedical concept, and is concerned with biological inferences. At face value this appears to be both a logical and sensible approach towards identifying trends in disease occurrence, populations at risk, possible preventative strategies and new therapies. However, crucial to this endeavour is the definition of **disease**, and as a corollary to this **illness, sickness** and **health**. What do epidemiologists mean by these terms? Are their conceptualisations the same as those of other health professionals and the lay public? The hegemony of medicine in epidemiology has ensured that the latter's approach to these conceptualisations is based largely on the models of Western medicine. This is despite epidemiology's attested concern with factors beyond the biological in the causation of disease.

Health: what is it?

Until relatively recently, health was referred to rather negatively as the absence of disease. Attempts to measure this concept are problematic, and indices of health status are usually based upon deviations from health, i.e. ill health. Although much has been written concerning this subject over the last 20 years (for example see Elinson, 1974; Sackett *et al.*, 1977; Headey *et al.* 1985), a definition for health remains elusive.

In clinical terms, health may be defined as the absence of disease, but two problems attach here. Firstly, in certain circumstances abnormal physiological or functional findings may be present in the absence of any discernible disease process. For example, a high concentration of serum cholesterol may be noted during screening of a seemingly healthy young man, or glucose may be found in the urine of a middle-aged woman who shows no other signs of diabetic pathology. Secondly, disease or physiological status do not fully embrace the image of health which most people hold. Other factors – social, psychological and cosmological – are all involved in perceptions of health. In other words, normality itself is a relative and judgemental concept (Mischler, 1981).

The World Health Organisation (1985) specified that health is 'a state of complete physical, mental and social well-being and not merely the absence of disease and infirmity'. The operationalisation of this definition has taxed observers ever since, although it has spearheaded the search for a broader more positive concept of health (Seedhouse, 1986). As Blaxter (1990) points out, such definitions are not new, echoing as they do the Galenian concepts of equilibrium and the Platonic model of health as harmony of the body's processes. Many of the respondents in her study of health and lifestyles identified with the WHO definition, conceptualising health as a relative state which was notably influenced by ageing. Such 'positive health' may ensue from many sources: 'the ability to cope with stressful situations, the maintenance of a strong social-support system,... high morale and life satisfaction,... and even levels of physical fitness as well as physical health' (Bowling, 1991, p. 7). This latter aspect is well portrayed in Crawford's exposition on healthism and social control (1984). He contends that Americans in general, and women in particular, conceptualise health as the control of their physical bodies, which is achieved through dieting and exercise.

Health, then, is not merely the absence of disease as conceptualised in the biomedical model, which epidemiology follows. The definition of disease does, however, fall more closely into the accepted philosophy and ideology of the scientific medicine adopted by practitioners in the Western world.

Disease – the medical perspective

Rene Descartes' treatise *The Passions of the Soul* (1649) has played a major role in shaping medical ideology. By proposing that the body and the soul are separate, Cartesian dualism legitimated the study of these two realms by distinctive disciplines. The body became the subject of the natural sciences and thence medicine, while the soul remained the province of the humanities. Thus biology was freed to pursue mechanistic theories of physiology and pathology in an era when natural science was developing the methods for investigating just such matters. This dualism also legitimated the 'reduction' of complex phenomena associated with the soul or mind into entities to be explained by, or in terms of, material causes. Increasingly, therefore, problems of the body were explained without any reference to psychological or sociocultural factors. The Flexner Report (1910) crystallised these sentiments by recognising the dominance of research-oriented scientific medicine as underpinned by a thorough training in biological and laboratory sciences. This report provided a model for future medical training both in the USA and in Europe (Turner, 1992).

The Cartesian mind/body split and the developing power of biological technology thus combined to construct a particular medical system – biomedicine. The basic premises of the Western medical perspective have been ascribed the following characteristics: scientific rationality; objectivity; quantitative measurement; and the concept of diseases as entities (Helman, 1990). Despite recent challenges to the supposed distinction between science and non-science (Kuhn, 1970), the dominant model of philosophical thought, which continues to shape the values and assumptions of biomedicine, is scientific rationality. That is (ostensibly anyway), the phenomena relating to health and sickness must be subjected to testing and verification under objective, empirical and controlled conditions. From thence they are translated into clinical facts, whose cause and effect await discovery. In this system phenomena which are readily measured and observed (for example, serum bilirubin concentrations or the size and distribution of skin lesions) are attributed greater 'reality' than other phenomena, such as anxiety, which are less amenable to quantitative measurements. These objective and verifiable clinical facts form the basis of consensus diagnoses which may be universally applied.

Ill health in medical terms is thus largely based on demonstrable physical changes in the body's structure or function. These changes are measured and then compared with a range of 'normal' physiological values. Each disease entity has certain recognisable characteristics that identify it, and such diseases are assumed to be 'universal in form and content' (Fabrega and Silver, 1973). The medical position is neatly encapsulated by a quotation from Lewis Thomas (1979, p. 168), a respected researcher: 'For every disease there is a single key mecha-

nism that dominates all others. If one can find it and think one's way
around it, one can control the disorder. In short I believe that the major
diseases of human beings have become approachable biological puz-
zles, ultimately solvable'. For medicine therefore, disease implies an
abnormality of structure/function, the need for correction, and the idea
that abnormalities are undesirable (Dingwall, 1976). Since conventional epidemiology is also grounded in scientific rationality its definition of disease also espouses these principles.

The making social of disease

Cassell (1976) has suggested that 'illness' is what a patient who goes
to the doctor is feeling, and 'disease' is what the person comes away
from the doctor's surgery with. Or as Eisenberg (1977, p. 11) puts it:
'patients suffer "illnesses", physicians diagnose and treat "diseases"'.
In the above discussion, disease is portrayed as deeply entrenched
within a medical arena. In this version of reality, diseases are in a sense
created through a professional discourse which is shaped and governed by its mentor – natural science. For other disciplines and for the
lay public a different set of beliefs and assumptions may inform the
framework around which health and ill health are constructed. The
ontological inheritance of sickness, illness and disease lies mainly
within three other disciplines – psychology, sociology and anthropology. Each has its own perspective, but the latter two disciplines have
run a somewhat similar course.

Psychology

A number of **psychological** theories have been postulated to understand the way in which people explain their own experience and
behaviour. Social learning theories assume that the learning experience of childhood shapes adult explanations. For example, Rotter's
locus of control construct (1966) suggests that those with consistent
experiences in childhood site control within themselves, and therefore
within their own actions, while those with inconsistent childhood
experiences believe that their own actions are irrelevant, and luck or
fate are deterministic. In contrast, social cognition purports that people make reality, i.e. incoming signals are interpreted in the light of
our own model of the world (Neisser, 1966). Developing this further,
personal construct theory (Kelly, 1966) views people as scientists who
continually test and modify their hypothesised world against reality.

Although personal construct theory credits individuals with more
sophisticated thinking, it is ultimately limited. Understanding and
explaining the world is more dialectic – it is a constant dynamic

between person-constructs-reality and reality-constructs-person (Buss, 1979). Dialectic explanations of illness and health operate in two domains, that of individual subjectivity and that of social and cultural inter-subjectivity. The explanation is derived not so much from the individual as from sets of ideas embedded in an ideological framework. Such theory posits the existence of explanations both inside and outside the person. By definition, such explanations will be shaped by social and cultural forces, as well as by the cognition of the individual. Herzlich (1973), describing such a model, suggests three personae for illness: illness as 'destroyer', illness as 'occupation' and illness as 'liberation'. These images are properties of both individuals and culture. While dialectically informed approaches undoubtedly offer a more sophisticated analysis, psychological theories in general take little cognisance of the subtle complexities of human nature, and obscure the significance of culture.

Sociology

Talcott Parsons (1951) first directed the attention of **sociology** to health and sickness by proposing a sick role. For Parsons the sick role is a form of deviance legitimised by both society in general and the 'healer' in specific. Four components can be recognised: exemption from normal social activities; exemption from responsibility for the condition; acknowledgement of the sick role as undesirable; and an expectation that competent help would be sought. By this model society controls the deviance of illness by the assignment of approved roles both to ill people and to those that care for them. This theory of societal action posits that particular social institutions govern people's behaviour and beliefs – structural functionalism.

In contrast, dominance theorists argue that the socially sedimented beliefs inherent in this model are not functional, but instead operate as a system of social control (Zola, 1972).

Both these approaches – functionalism and dominance theory – assume that people's understandings are constructed for them. Dingwall (1976), however, argues that reality is actively constructed by all social groups. The explanatory models of lay people should therefore be recognised as functional within their own domain. Similarly, Friedson (1970) highlights the importance of the lay referral system, and suggests that 'it is lay culture, and not the professional values of the physician, which defines the meaning of illness in the social context' (Turner, 1987, p. 45). Although these ideas do not preclude that, in part, knowledge is constructed for people, a wider notion of thoughtful and purposive analysis is embraced.

Anthropology

Nascent **anthropological** explanations of illness and health were obscured by a preoccupation with medical systems (rather than beliefs), and by distinctions between 'primitive' and 'civilised' systems. However, as more ecological theories were formulated the importance of considering political and social influences alongside biological and environmental factors was appreciated. This eclectic outlook allowed explanatory systems concerning health and illness to be reconciled with the prevailing ideologies and societies in which they operated. It also recognised the significance of medical pluralism. Medical pluralism refers to the coexistence of several systems of health therapy within a society. Some commentators consider that today the medical systems of most communities are characterised by pluralism (Young, 1982).

Anthropology thus began to realise a number of frameworks through which health and sickness might be articulated. These included Valabrega's account of exogenous and endogenous causality (1962); Foster's distinction of personalistic (where illness is derived from a motivated intervention by another person, or being) and naturalistic (where illness results from nature) systems (1976); and Leslie's comprehensive classification, which construes health/illness with mechanistic characteristics (smooth running/breakdown), equilibrium elements (balance/disharmony), and ethical components (the good man/the transgressor) (Stainton-Rogers, 1991).

Further exploration of the concepts of sickness, illness and disease can be found in the work of Good, Kleinman and Young, which is rooted in a cognitive approach based on semantics (the meaning of language). Kleinman (1978, p. 88), developing Fabrega (1974) and Eisenberg (1977), proposes disease as denoting 'a malfunctioning... of biological and/or psychological processes. Illness on the other hand signifies the experience of disease... and the societal reaction to disease'. Further, Good and Good (1981) developed the concept of semantic illness networks, which encompassed linked ideas and definitions that enabled the explanation not only of biological reality, but the moral, social and religious aspects also. Similarly Kleinman proposed explanatory models (EMs) as containing the knowledge which people invoked when ill, and also the roles and norms of conduct to be adopted. These models act therefore not only as explanations to those who are ill, but also as templates for becoming and being ill. In other words, EMs are both models of, and models for reality. Using Good's conception of semantic illness networks and his own model of EMs, Kleinman proposed the following schema to distinguish between and describe the concepts of disease, illness and sickness from an anthropological viewpoint:

- Disease: a malfunction in structure or function – a pathological state
- Illness: a person's perception and experience of socially devalued states
- Sickness: a blanket term covering both disease and illness

Other medical anthropologists have attempted to redefine a more eclectic interpretation of the human experience of ill health. Frankenberg (1980) and Young (1982) adopted a position which gave primacy to the social relations of sickness. While accepting the previous definitions of disease and illness, sickness became the **social recognition** of disease and illness (Frankenberg), or **a process** for socialising disease and illness (Young). Further, Hahn (1983) suggests the concept of suffering, which results from the interaction of illness (the ideas of patients), disease (the ideologies of biomedical practitioners) and disorder (the specific perspective of non-Western healers). These three ideologies are egalitarian and may exist in five different 'sites' in which the problem of suffering is localised – physical, personal, social, environmental and cosmological. Thus Hahn posits the idea of suffering as an abstract concept, whereas Scheper-Hughes and Lock (1987), taking a phenomenological approach, focus on the suffering person.

Stacey (1988, p. 142) proposes that **lay** ideas concerning why, when, and how misfortune enters people's lives are logical and valid in their own right, even if not consonant with biomedical science. Fundamental to any explanation of becoming ill and subsequently recovering is the concept of causality. One of the simplest frameworks for viewing causality categorises illnesses into those within the individual (endogenous) and those attributed to the world outside (exogenous). Within the first group the individual is deemed responsible for choices concerning sickness, and although such explanations have been most often described in pre-literate societies, psychoanalytical explanations of psychosomatic disease in Western societies and conditions such as *susto*, in South America, stress the individual's culpability. In contrast, exogenous theories attribute causality to fate or the influence of powerful others. Such explanations are said to be more common in Western societies, where the germ theory of disease predominates (Wilkinson, 1988).

Indeed, external causes (infection, poor working conditions, climate) were most frequently cited in a study of working class women in Aberdeen (Blaxter and Paterson, 1982). Although personal behaviour was recognised as a factor precipitating illness, it was not perceived as causal. The cause lay in the conditions in which the respondents were required to live. Similarly, Herzlich (1973) reported that illness among Parisians was construed as a result of an assault from outside, for example pollution or overcrowding. A study of the lay beliefs concerning the causality of colds and fevers (Helman, 1978) also emphasised the prominent role of a hostile world, beset with both natural (cold air, germs) and supernatural (devils, spirits) forces, in the aetiology of illness. This clear-cut dichotomous model was, however, expanded by Pill and Stott's studies of Welsh working class women (1982; 1985) which demonstrated three clusters of causal attribution. According to these authors, most people appear capable of holding a number of contradictory theories of causation at the same time (Pill and Stott, 1985). More recently they suggest that health and lifestyle behaviour are the result of a complex interplay of socio-demographic factors, understandings and barriers to action (Pill and Stott, 1987). Whilst Blaxter's survey (1990) also intimates that health and illness are constructed and rationalised in a wider framework of cultural discourses, themes and messages.

To summarise, a gradual trend towards a much richer tapestry of explanatory sympatricity is evident. Not only do alternative explanations of health and illness coexist and compete, but 'available' knowledge may vary in form, time and place, while different processes (for example, recovery, resistance and ageing) will entail different explanations. The biomedical model, although invoked to some extent, is a barren cake shorn of its icing. Individuals and collectives draw on multiple realities. A collage of ideologies, personal experience, religion, folk wisdom and social factors shapes explanations of health and illness. Consequently, courses of action and perceptions of personal control thereby become a synthesis of the social, circumstantial and environmental forces surrounding an individual. The reality is of people as 'clever weavers of stories... who create order out of chaos' (Stainton Rogers, 1991, p. 10).

SICKNESS – THE MOST APPROPRIATE PARADIGM?

The discussion above begins to unravel the different ways in which both academic disciplines and lay people conceptualise becoming and being sick. Despite moves towards a more biopsychosocial model (Engel, 1980), the medical focus remains on disease entities, while the humanities encapsulate a perspective where the sociocultural milieu of ill health is just as significant as any physiological or structural malfunctioning of the body. These differences assume particular importance in epidemiology, which, although based largely on biomedical precepts, also recognises the crucial role that social factors play in disease aetiology. The mechanisms through which epidemiology conceptualises such factors may, however, be problematic, and this will be further discussed below in the context of the medicalisation of the discipline.

As this chapter has developed it has become increasingly apparent that the biomedical model of disease could be expanded and enriched through a consideration of the lay perspective on health and illness, which has been revealed largely through anthropological study. If epidemiology is to gain a more thorough understanding of the social factors that affect disease, it will have to adopt a more sophisticated approach to the mechanisms through which such factors are constituted and act. It will be necessary to broaden the conceptualisations through, and by which, medicine's biological disease is recognised as society's sickness. This section continues to expand on the concept of sickness through a further consideration of who recognises sickness and how it is recognised. Epidemiology is often concerned with measuring the rate of ill health in different populations and attempting to determine the reasons for it, and thereby the most effective methods for preventing or treating ill health. How sickness is construed, and how and by whom this construction is recognised, is therefore of crucial importance to the pursuit of the subject.

Who recognises sickness?

It is apparent from the foregoing that several different disciplines have an interest in the concepts of disease and sickness, and that widely different approaches to the conceptualisation of these terms may be invoked according to the epistemology[1] of the subject concerned. Notwithstanding this, there is also a wide range to the interpretations which may be applied according to theoretical positions within disciplines. This is particularly obvious within sociology and anthropology, where approaches range between explanations that are founded on structural functionalism (for example Hahn (1983)) and, at the other end of the spectrum, explanations such as those of Scheper-Hughes and Lock (1987), which encompass an interpretative stance rooted in phenomenology. In addition, although biomedical explanations are essentially embedded in a rational framework, the practice of biomedicine sometimes belies its supposedly scientific character

1 Epistemology concerns an understanding of the sources and processes of knowledge.

(Rhodes, 1990). This loosening of the scientific bond is particularly striking in chronic illness, when the interpretation of theory and practice is 'left much to the discretion of individual clinicians... [reflecting] personal biography,... age, subspecialty or institutional affiliation' (Lock and Gordon, 1988, p. 12). However, it is perhaps with those outside the healthcare professions that the framework which both categorises sickness and explains why certain individuals become ill at certain times assumes its most varied and changeable format.

In this somewhat confusing area there are three principal 'actors' who may recognise sickness – self, lay others and professional others. 'Recognition' in this sense means both a conscious construction of a category (sickness) which is matched against previous experience, and a legitimisation of that category in a social world. Within the medical, and thus the epidemiological, framework the recognition of ill health is ostensibly clear-cut and dependent upon the demonstration of physical signs or symptoms consonant with the agreed definitions of a particular disease entity. If such markers of disease are not present, then the patient even if continuing to feel 'ill', is told that there is nothing wrong. The presence of objectively demonstrable changes in structure and function are therefore usually integral to the medical category 'disease'. Furthermore, within the confines of the medical encounter disease is usually synonymous with sickness. However, in certain instances, which will be discussed later, obvious physical signs may be ignored, or at least not acknowledged by doctors.

For a sociologist such as Twaddle (1981, p. 112) the question of who recognises sickness is equally clear-cut: 'The ill person is judged by others to be sick'. In the first instance, these others refer to the laity, friends, family members etc. The health professional subsequently 'converts the sickness from one based on illness into one based on disease, or failing to make the conversion, rejects the designation of the patient as sick' (Twaddle, 1981, p. 112). According to the health professional this person is not sick, but what is his position with regard to family and friends? If he was sick before, why is he sick no longer? The critical point here is whether it is biomedicine or society that recognises sickness. Is society's recognition of sickness dependent on a professional healer's legitimisation? In some cases this appears so, but since medical systems are in themselves social constructs the ultimate recourse does in fact seem to be with society.

The question of self-recognition of sickness is also problematic. Here Hahn's idea (1983) of an overall concept of suffering subsuming sickness as one referent in a system where disease, illness and disorder operate for different actors in a different time and space is more helpful than a simple notion of sickness as the socialisation of disease. The sense of individuals being active, creating the world in which they live, is important here. Constructs such as sickness may be taken as already defined, or modified versions may be created both by the individual and those around him.

How is sickness recognised?

If the analysis above is correct in its conclusion that sickness is recognised by society, then two possible aspects of that recognition are noteworthy: sickness as a social role and sickness as a moral category. For Talcott Parsons (1951) sickness was a form of deviant behaviour which required legitimisation and social control. However, many criticisms of this model have been put forward (Turner, 1987). The sick role fails to accommodate chronic illness; fails to disentangle the conflicts between doctors and patients; ignores the lay referral system; and does not distinguish between patient role and sick role. As Turner notes (1987, p. 46), 'not all sick people are patients, and not all patients are sick people'. Nevertheless, the conception of sickness as a social category is useful. Many cultures allow for a temporary respite from social obligations under the label of sickness. For example, Morsy (1978) describes 'possession sickness' in women as a socially acceptable way to avoid certain social obligations. Becoming 'possessed' enables the woman to perhaps avoid an arranged marriage. Locker (1983) has argued against the idea of sickness as a deviant state. He suggests that sickness is 'a symbolic ordering of given events by the application of a label. It is a social state created by human evaluation'. He draws the distinction between illness behaviours and being allocated into a social state of illness. Making the point that sickness labels are neither ethically neutral nor value-free, he suggests that definitions of sickness are therefore social constructs and, as such, are moral constructs.

Despite the above, however, the clarification of the concept of sickness, and thus how and by who it is recognised, is far from complete. Is sickness a behaviour? A social state? Or a meaning/explanation? It is to these issues that a more perspicacious epidemiology should be applying itself.

PERSPECTIVES ON NORMALITY AND ABNORMALITY

The biomedical view

In all epidemiological studies it is necessary sooner or later to define whether a subject is abnormal (in traditional parlance, diseased) or normal (disease-free). Working within the confines of the biomedical model *sensu stricto* this should not cause too many problems, although decisions about what is normal are more difficult among the general population than in a selected group such as hospitalised patients. Normality is defined by reference to particular physical and biochemical parameters, for example weight, blood count, respiratory rate, concentration of hormones, absence of cellular changes and blood pressure. For many of these measurements there is a normal range below or above which disease may be indicated. If measurements fall within the normal range the individual is declared healthy. Thus if on a routine health screening a young woman is found to have a diastolic blood pressure of over 100 mm Hg she will be recalled for a further series of measurements, and if the finding is confirmed she will be recommended a course of treatment. However, the relationship between abnormal physiological or structural findings and disease is not always straightforward. Even where the objective tenets of science act as the standard for decisions concerning who is and is not diseased, certain difficulties may arise.

Much of the medical definition of disease is based on the type of precise measurements which emanate from the biological and physical sciences. Medicine in its turn will therefore be bounded by the potential constraints which accompany such measurements. The quality of measurements is an important consideration. Within the scientific framework measurements need to be shown as both **valid** and **reliable**. Validity (or accuracy) refers to the degree to which the measurement corresponds to the true state (see also Chapter 1). Reliability concerns the extent to which repeated measurements align with each other. It is not difficult to understand that validity and reliability are more easily determined for 'hard' measurements (perhaps serum albumin concentration or level of thyrotoxine, which may be compared with some accepted scientific standard) than for 'soft' parameters, such as distress or emotional well-being, for which science and Western medicine have no accepted 'gold standards'. This epitomises biomedicine, which defines its diseases through the demonstration of a deviation from normal values as characterised by objectivity and rational measurement. In this model, if diseases are not reduced to a series of empirical measurements difficulties in their recognition will ensue. Where no physical standards of validity exist, such as would be the case for measuring nausea or pain, attempts are still made to rationalise measurements using scales constructed through the use of standardised patient questionnaires. Bowling (1991) provides an excellent account of such scales used in measuring the quality of life.

Variation in measurements may also play a part in the results that are obtained from a clinical test. This variation might lead to erroneous conclusions being drawn from the data. Two sources of variation may be identified – measurement variation and biological variation. The former occurs through inconsistencies in the performance of the people and instruments used in making the measurements. Both random (or chance) and systematic (or biased) errors may occur (see Chapter 1 for a fuller discussion of these concepts). Biological phenomena are not consistent, and variation in measurements may arise either within individuals or among individuals. Thus measurements of blood pressure in the same person over three consecutive days may provide three different readings. The difficulty is in deciding which measure, if any is the 'true' reading.

This raises the issue of what is abnormal. In considering this, clinicians have recourse to examine the way in which a particular measure, say serum creatinine concentration, is distributed among a population. A graph of the proportion of people exhibiting certain values may be plotted (a frequency distribution). If there are sharply defined boundaries between the distributions of measurements for normal people and those for abnormal people, then the classification of the particular condition associated with the measurement is relatively simple. For example, Fletcher *et al.* (1988) provide the example of the clear separation between the two distribution curves for people with normal and abnormal glutathione metabolism. Such clear-cut separations are, however, rare, and very often the values for the diseased overlap with those of the normal population. Difficulties in deciding on a cut-off point above or below which disease may be defined then ensue.

Very often, clinical medicine will adopt a statistical approach and consider abnormality as something which occurs infrequently. Normal is usual and abnormal is unusual. However, this may create ambiguities: for example, a particularly low or indeed high result from a test may be unusual, but it does not necessarily indicate disease. Also, some patients who from clinical examination are clearly diseased have 'normal' laboratory tests; such is the case in normocalcaemic hypothyroidism or aseptic meningitis. Sackett *et al.* (1991) provide further examples of the different ways in which normality has been defined in clinical medicine and the problems that have arisen.

Another difficulty is that even where such objective measures as blood pressure are used in the definition of abnormality there may remain controversy as to what the normal range should be. This may result from a genuine lack of knowledge concerning normal ranges in particular patients. For example, as increasing numbers of babies born prematurely survived it became necessary to determine new ranges of parameters that accurately reflected their immature physiological status. In addition, questions as to how rapidly such infants adapted to and regained a physiological status comparable with a baby born at term needed to be answered. Is a two-week-old baby born at 26 weeks gestation the same as a day-old baby born at 28 weeks gestation?

The above discussion illustrates that although the biomedical definitions of normality and abnormality appear straightforward, difficulties may arise. Those same objective scientific measurements that are integral to the model bring their own characteristic problems. For epidemiology, some important points emerge. If the biomedical definitions of abnormality and normality are assumed, then the same difficulties constraining their use within medicine will apply equally to epidemiology. In particular, it is evident that the type of population – in the hospital or the community, young or old – that is selected in any attempt to define normal or abnormal will influence the conclusions drawn. In addition, estimates of the relative prevalence of abnormalities will also be affected by the population studied. What is also clear to any astute observer is that scientific medicine is not the sole basis by which normal and abnormal health are defined in our own or other populations.

The sociocultural view

The account above explained the basis through which Western medicine comes to conclusions concerning what is normal and therefore by extension what constitutes ill health and the possible need for intervention. Another viewpoint holds that although disease may be seen as a biological deviation, what is normal and abnormal is a social and moral judgement. It is the prevalent social values that define what is acceptable and therefore 'normal'. As Jones and Moon (1987, p. 5) note, 'in contrast to the biomedical notion of universal generic diseases, the social view accepts that what constitutes disease can vary temporally, culturally and indeed, geographically'.

Several situations may arise through which social or cultural factors may influence how normality is perceived both by healthcare professionals and by lay people. Two main categories may be discerned: instances where the definition of abnormality arises through a medical discourse (albeit couched within a social framework), and instances where abnormality is largely defined by significant 'others' not connected with the delivery of healthcare. In the first category biomedicine is ostensibly taken as the framework through which decisions are made. However, in particular circumstances confusion arises concerning the boundaries of normality and abnormality. Two examples will be provided: the phenomenon of 'disease without illness' and the situation when practitioners ignore the objective evidence of biomedicine in their construction of a patient's illness.

In many instances a person may not feel 'ill' and yet because of modern medicine's emphasis on diagnostic technology may be considered abnormal. Examples of such cases include hypertension, elevated liver enzymes or carcinomas. This 'disease without illness' is both the rationale but also the dilemma of screening programmes (see also Chapter 6). Where it is clear that such abnormal results presage serious or imminent ill health then the recognition of these early signs may be life-saving. In these cases it is clear to the doctor that although the patient is not currently sick it is extremely likely that they will become so and this information should be imparted together with a mutually acceptable plan for any intervening treatment.

However, in many instances the significance of the abnormal result is less clear. Such has been the recent controversy concerning screening for serum cholesterol levels as an indicator of potential heart disease. Although initial studies indicated that people with a raised cholesterol level were at greater risk (Kannel *et al.*, 1962) subsequent more in-depth research, which combined the results of several clinical trials (meta-analysis) raised doubts, and moreover indicated that treatment with cholesterol-lowering drugs was associated with an elevated mortality (Oliver *et al.*, 1980). The difficulty here is that with insufficient or faulty knowledge biomedicine cannot accurately predict the future. For some practitioners such individuals are abnormal; for others they may be normal. Whichever way, there is a moral dilemma as to what patients should be told about their prognoses.

Undoubtedly Western medicine has an enviable reputation for its ability to diagnose and treat a wide range of acute illnesses. However, the biomedical model and indeed the entire cultural and ideological persona of scientific medicine is thrown into disarray by the existence of chronic illnesses, untreatable conditions, or phenomena such as pain which so obviously have dimensions beyond the purely physical. Frankenberg (1992, p. 74) suggests that chronicity is more challenging than acute illness because 'its persistent presence is a theological embarrassment to religion, a scientific embarrassment to medicine, and an economic embarrassment to state and civil society'.

Placed in this type of situation, then, medical practitioners may sometimes fail to acknowledge the biological implications of disease in an attempt to socially reconstruct their patient's illness. Such a case is described by Silverman (1987) in his discourse analysis of the interactions between doctors and the parents of children who may require heart surgery. Some of the children had Down's syndrome and others did not. Two interesting points emerge. Firstly, non-Down's syndrome children are described by the doctor as 'well', for example 'a well little girl who's got a heart murmur'. The mother contests this definition of wellness – after all if she has been referred to the clinic how can her child be well? Thus, despite the evidence of biological abnormality – disease – these children are constructed by the clinical encounter as well. Since many of these children will undergo surgery it is difficult to understand when and how they become sick – perhaps on entry to hospital? Secondly, Down's syndrome children are manoeuvred into a social rather than a medical discourse. Again by the tenets of biomedicine these children have demonstrable abnormalities in lung and heart function, but there is a reluctance to operate and the child's illness remains as such. Illness is not translated into sickness by the doctor, since once translated further medical intervention may be morally and ethically demanded. It is difficult to know how the parents perceive their child – is she healthy? Probably not.

The examples above illustrate occasions when healthcare professionals have recourse to either question or reinterpret biomedical evidence in their classification of the normal and abnormal. This activity occurs to a much greater extent among those people who are outside the healthcare professions. At the beginning of this chapter some insights were provided into the nature and importance of lay explanations of health and illness, which not unnaturally run parallel with similar conceptions concerning normality. The diagnosis of abnormality is not restricted to the medical domain. To recognise abnormality it is first necessary to have noticed some departure from normality, with the integral presumption that various standards that characterise normal exist. Lewis (1993, p. 100) contends that such standards are set both individually and by society: individually, since each of us knows the extent and boundaries of our own body's functioning, and culturally because society sets the boundaries to expectations and 'establishes criteria of approval, and normality'. Normal function then becomes relative to circumstances and to individuals.

A particularly noteworthy example of this is provided by Scheper-Hughes (1978) in her study 'Saints, scholars and schizophrenics – Madness and badness in Western Ireland'. Epidemiological data show that psychiatric hospitalisation and the diagnosis of schizophrenia were particularly common in Ireland in the 1960s and 1970s. Indeed, on census day in 1971, 2% of males in Western Ireland were in a mental hospital (O'Hare and Walsh, 1971). In addition, epidemiological surveys have demonstrated a statistical association between such afflictions and male sex, peripheral agriculture, depopulation and celibacy. This 'unique epidemiological profile' suggests that sociocultural factors may have a major role to play in the diagnosis and treatment of mental illness in this community.

Through an exploration of the community definitions of normality and abnormality and the sociological milieu in which they prevail, Scheper-Hughes attempts to reveal the mechanisms through which both society and medicine collude in the construction of this sickness. She notes how in rural Irish villages, although 'saints' (quiet but eccentric individuals) are tolerated and even cultivated, those who 'violate the strong sanctions against expressions of sexuality, aggression, and disrespectful subordination to parental or religious authority' are perceived as non-conformists and 'as prime candidates for the mental hospital' (Scheper-Hughes 1978, p. 74). Thus a narrow definition of normal behaviour, coupled with the types of hospital facility that were available, created a particular circumstance that enabled large numbers of young bachelors to be labelled as mentally ill and institutionalised. Although not trained in psychiatry it was clear to the researcher that these inmates were alienated and seeking some respite for their condition. 'If not diseased in a medical sense, the patients were dis-eased in a sociological sense' (Scheper-Hughes, 1978, p. 68).

Many other instances of the cultural construction of normality and abnormality both within and without the medical discourse could be cited. Indeed, although sociologists and anthropologists frequently portray biomedicine as a discrete and bounded entity it would be superficial to claim that these two worlds, lay and professional, do not overlap and merge. Doctors and epidemiologists are part of society too! Distinctions between the normal and abnormal may be blurred according to the particular condition under scrutiny, the ideology of the physician to whom the complaint is presented, and the specific sociocultural context in which they are working.

THE MEDICALISATION OF EPIDEMIOLOGY

Much of the foregoing has hinted that some of the problems and unresolved dilemmas of epidemiology may be attributed to the discipline's strong association with medicine. In this context this section will explore the history of scientific medicine and its relationship with epidemiology in order to confront some of the assumptions on which both subjects are based. This will lead to an examination of disease classification within biomedicine and how this may influence the framework through which epidemiology is pursued.

The way to scientific medicine

The epistemology of biomedicine provides the basis for explaining the medical perspective on disease. The framework of medieval medicine rested on the humoral theory of disease deriving from Hippocrates, Empedocles and Galen. This theory posited the world in terms of four elements (fire, earth, air and water) and four qualities (blood, phlegm, yellow bile and black bile). The conceptualisation was of the body in equilibrium, with illness occurring when an imbalance in humoral activity occurred. This form of medicine continued to be practised until the latter part of the 18th century, although social and theoretical developments were gradually invoking major changes in both philosophy and practice.

The Galenic legacy was first challenged in 1543 by Vesalius, whose treatise on human dissections pre-empted the emergence of pathological anatomy and a growing concern with science. Increasingly, vitalism was being overtaken by a mechanistic philosophy. Thus, instead of nature ordering events through the harmony of God's plans, the world was conceived as a machine which, if reduced to its component parts, could be explained by the laws of mathematics. Cartesian dualism (Descartes, 1649) which separated the material from the spiritual world, the body from the spirit, both shaped and yet allowed for such radical changes in philosophical thought. Corporeal Man could be governed by mechanics and investigated by the methods of science, while Man's spiritual being, his emotions, values and feelings, remained with the soul. Thus the fundamental task during the enlightenment was the separation of nature from its metaphysical and spiritual connections. Nature was considered to be orderly and predictable, the key to the universe being logic, not spiritual meaning. Natural science developed from the assertion that nature was autonomous from cosmos, society and culture, human consciousness, and particular time and space. Reductionism (the philosophy that the ultimate explanation of a phenomenon is best provided by analysing or dissecting down to its separate parts) dominated the study of the body and medicine.

In consequence a general trend towards empiricism evolved, since only things that were measurable were considered scientific. This increasing empiricism was particularly influenced by Francis Bacon and Robert Boyle, and was notable in the clinical methods of Sydenham and Locke. Biomedicine thus evolved through the emancipation of scientific enlightenment and the regression of the Church's proscription of human dissection.

The move towards reductionism was further boosted towards the end of the 19th century and was particularly evident in laboratory medicine, which focused not on the patient as a whole, but on tissues or even cells. In order to pursue such studies an even greater input from the natural sciences was required. More importantly however, the clinical diagnosis became centred on such science through the use of tests and technological procedures. Pasteur's germ theory of disease and the work of Koch (see Chapter 1) further underwrote the scientific approach and spawned two important ideas – specific aetiology and magic bullets. The former theory posited that each disease had a single, specific and objective cause, while the latter embraced the idea that such causes could be selectively destroyed. Through these developments the vision of the whole body was discarded, analysis replaced synthesis, and physicalism weakened vitalism. As Hahn and Kleinman (1983, p. 307) put it 'Biomedicine became a paradigmatic exemplar of these materialistic tendencies'. According to Foucault (1973) modern medicine was born when the 'medical gaze' was brought to bear on the body, and a recognition of what was individual and what was abnormal emerged. The clinico-pathological correlate, hinging critically on post mortem examination, was the linchpin of this new medicine. Symptoms and histories related by the patient were interpreted by the doctor in conjunction with the signs from clinical examination to infer the presence of the lesion.

The development of modern medicine must therefore be viewed as resulting as much from changes in the socio-political environment as from scientific progress. This apart, its model of reasoning remains deductive, and its operationalisation essentially reductionist. Biological reductionism is the dominant model of philosophical thought that shapes the basic values and assumptions of biomedicine today. Indeed, despite recent challenges to the supposed distinction between science and non-science (Kuhn, 1970), the natural science paradigm remains dominant in medicine. Taylor (1985, p. 6) suggests that this persistence is not grounded in a belief that science produces 'better' knowledge. He conjectures that the image of science, embodying as it does a disengagement of subject from object, is deeply attractive to the human ego. 'In short the epistemological weaknesses [of the natural science paradigm] are more than made up for by its moral appeal' (Taylor, 1985, p. 6).

Further, Gordon (1988) considers that many of the assumptions salient to science appear in biomedical discourse and practice. By exploring the veracity of the claim that biomedicine and science are autonomous from society she exposes a triadic support between these two and the concept of the individual. Individualism, she asserts, is a dominant and prized value of Western society which has much in common with science, and by implication with biomedicine. The philosophy that these paradigms are free from the constructs of society and culture cannot therefore in her view be supported. Neither science nor biomedicine are free from cultural values. Gordon thus builds an eloquent argument which furthers the original challenges of those who suggest that both science and medicine are essentially social enterprises (Latour and Woolgar, 1979; Mulkay, 1979; Wright and Treacher, 1982). Navarro (1980, p. 540) pursues this theme using a Marxist perspective. He believes that biomedicine was not created by scientific discovery, but rather by the 'victory of the bourgeoisie which established that positivist conception of science and medicine'.

In the face of these arguments, the image of modern medicine, based as it is on an objective, pure science devoid of moral or ideological bias, becomes somewhat flawed. The adoption of science as the métier for Western medicine can be seen as part of the mores of a developing capitalist society which prized individualism and materialism, themselves inextricably linked to naturalistic science. It is not just a matter of ideologies, however. The day-to-day practice of biomedicine belies its supposedly scientific character. Science may ostensibly be applied to medicine, but it is certainly modified, or even radically transformed, by the unique perspectives of the actors involved. Thus, although biological reductionism is offered as the hallmark of biomedicine, its practice often differs significantly from this standard rhetoric (Rhodes, 1990). Indeed, recent attempts by government bodies to rationalise practice are witness to this. The production of scientific guidelines or protocols and the search for an explication of the decision-making processes of doctors are both efforts to neutralise the intuitive aspects of practice and to remove the physician's personal power and private magic.

The classification of disease

Classification depends on the recognition of differences and similarities between cases. Unfortunately, the biomedical model of disease classification has been uncritically espoused on the basis that since it was scientific, it was objective and value-free. The perceived exclusion of social or moral judgements in its construction was further evidence of its unbiased character and thus worthy status as a universal standard against which other lesser classifications should be compared. Dingwall (1992) remarks on how the study of classificatory systems in medicine has been neglected. For many years social scientists and anthropologists have examined and compared the medical systems of other cultures, frequently referring them back to biomedicine. Serious analyses of Western medicine as a cultural system in its own right, as just another ethnomedicine, have been singularly lacking.

However, the concepts, theories and models of biomedicine are not solely embedded in scientific rationality, but are part of a wider perspective. Epidemiology is wrestling to free itself from the old model of one agent/one disease which characterised the work of the early pioneers of scientific medicine. The social and environmental influences that affect the distribution of disease in a population do not lend themselves readily to mathematical models. Stallones (1980) draws attention to the fact that many epidemiologists are physicians and as such have become habituated into the biomedical mode. They are 'deeply imprinted and reluctant to accept that most biomedical research is irrelevant to the solution of community health problems' (Stallones, 1980, p. 76). For them, disease classifications which evolved through the practice of clinical medicine have become the norm, and other systems, such as those based on environmental or social groupings, are ignored. Also embedded within both lay and medical discourses is the notion that diseases are entities, and this is encapsulated in the concept of their supposed 'natural history'. Sydenham, the 17th century English physician, purported this idea by likening diseases to growing seeds, which show a regular pattern of development and progress. He wrote, 'All diseases then ought to be reduc'd to certain and determinate kinds, with the same exactness as we see it done by botanic writers in their treatises of plants' (Sydenham, 1742, p. iv).

The social construction of disease confronts this biological view of nature producing disease in a constant and distinct way. Diseases are not independent entities – things – but a 'selection of attributes characteristically shown by people who fall ill in this way' (Lewis, 1993, p. 95). Diseases do not exist in nature: there are micro-organisms and there are human hosts, but diseases are 'produced by the conceptual schemes imposed on the natural world by human beings, which value some states of the body and disvalue others' (Dingwall, 1992, p. 165). Biological changes are a material fact, but it is the significance of those changes that matters. For example, physiological ageing is an undeniable aspect of the life course, and growing old in Western society is conceived as a problem, almost a disease. However, for the inhabitants of the Trobriand Islands the ravages of middle age in men are reconceptualised through a cultural strategy associated with *Kula* magic[2]. In this context, the reality of ageing bodies is denied

---

2   The *Kula* is an elaborate form of gift exchange which occurs among the

through a symbolic elaboration associated with a ritual (Spencer, 1990).

Pertinent here also is Friedson's contention (1970) that medical practitioners are the architects of medical knowledge and thus gain the power to construct knowledge for others. In particular, Taussig (1980) has suggested that biomedicine 'reproduces a political ideology in the guise of a science of (apparently) real things'. Both Taussig and Young (1980) have argued that such reification constructs a particular version of reality and colludes in the reproduction of social power relations in capitalist society. As one doctor in a study by Posner (1984) of diabetic clinics in London told him, 'diabetes is what I say it is'.

The biomedical model of classification is therefore just one view of the world, which for the most part neglects the sociocultural context in which the majority of illnesses are experienced. This narrow classification is based on collecting information about a particular constellation of symptoms, which for clinical medicine represents disease. If epidemiology relies entirely on this type of model it will be in grave danger of ignoring those factors that are most important in the prediction and prevention of sickness. The preceding section provided some examples of how normality and abnormality and thus health and ill health might be defined from different viewpoints.

Disease classification systems form part of this process of recognition and acknowledgement of the abnormal. Western classifications, far from remaining static representations of some universal truth, change with current knowledge and the revision of standards. Indeed, as has been noted earlier, scientific ideals are much less evidenced in practice than in rhetoric. Even when confined to the medical systems of seemingly similar countries, such as France, Germany and the UK, fundamental differences in classifications and treatments of diseases are only too evident. Payer (1989) describes one such instance when a disease in one country is even considered as particularly good health in another! British and North American physicians are only too delighted if their patients have a diastolic blood pressure below 70 mm Hg, believing that this endows them with a low risk of future cardiovascular disease. However, in Germany doctors define hypotension as a disease with particular symptoms which require treatment. There are problems then even with allegedly clear-cut medical classifications.

Trobriand Islanders in the Western Pacific and was first described by Malinowski (1922). Those who sail to exchange gifts are in business and the ritual is a form of internal prestige among the men, not all of whom take part. *Kula* networks reinforce rank and power, and the exchange of gifts creates and sustains relations of inequality.

For psychology and psychiatry these difficulties are doubly manifest. Of particular note are the attempts of psychiatry to apply universal classifications of mental illness across different cultures. Deprived of the measurable biological indices by which physical illness is diagnosed, psychiatry relies on the subjective opinion of the practitioner, who will compare the cluster of presenting symptoms with the typical 'textbook' case. Such diagnoses have been shown to be heavily influenced by the psychiatrist's original trainer (Kendell, 1975) and the variable format of the diagnostic categories themselves. The dramatic effect that influential opinion may have was shown in a classic experiment by Temerlin (1968). He demonstrated that information provided by an authoritative figure shortly before viewing a video of an actor trained to display normal behaviour greatly influenced the diagnosis that a group of psychologists came to following the viewing. Only 8% of a group that overheard a remark that the man was neurotic and psychotic pronounced him normal, whereas 100% of another audience who were fed the remark that the man was 'perfectly healthy' pronounced him so.

The view that diseases are entities and that primacy should be given to Western medical diagnostic and labelling systems is expressed by some psychiatrists. Kiev (1972) for example contends that conditions such as schizophrenia are fixed in form by humanity's biological nature, only conceding that the content of say, delusions, will vary according to the sociocultural context.

For epidemiology, the classification of disease, or in other words normal and abnormal, is central to its field of activities. By adopting a biomedical approach to disease classification two problems are evident. Firstly the hegemony of scientific medicine has created the idea that diseases are specific entities, things almost, which may only be defined through the methods and technologies of biological pathology. By focusing on dysfunction of the corporeal body, aspects of the mind are rendered secondary and unimportant to the genesis of illness. This preoccupation with the individual body, or in reality the organs and cells of the body, also stifles any realisation that wider macro-level factors, such as the environment or politics, may influence the prevalence or progress of illness at any particular time.

Secondly, the manifestation of many sicknesses particularly those of a psychological origin is crucially affected by the cultural context in which they occur. These sicknesses, indeed probably all sicknesses, cannot be adequately defined through the categories of Western societies. Kleinman (1987) notes how much cross-cultural research has been undertaken to illustrate that psychiatric illnesses are universal, and like other disorders can be detected through the use of standardised diagnostic techniques. He suggests that much of this research commits a 'category fallacy'. This occurs when a nosological category developed for one culture is reified (i.e. made into a 'thing' – see above) and then applied to people of other cultures. Thus Western categories of psychiatric disorder are imposed on cultures for which they lack validity. Categories of disorder are created in particular places and particular times, and to attempt to use these across cultures is meaningless. Kleinman provides the example of a psychiatrist from a non-Western society attempting to measure the prevalence of 'soul loss' in urban middle class Americans. As he notes (1987, p. 452), 'He would come up with prevalence data. But would such data be valid, inasmuch as the disorder soul loss has no coherence for middle class North Americans?'.

Challenging the medicalisation of epidemiology

The section above discusses how epidemiology has increasingly become dominated by the paradigm of biomedicine and the natural sciences, and how this has led to a particular conceptualisation of disease classification. This final section will describe an emerging challenge to medical epidemiology as witnessed by the efforts of **popular epidemiology**. This activity involves lay people in the collection of epidemiological data, which is interpreted in conjunction with experts in order to understand the epidemiology of disease. It thus involves processes which call on the types of lay knowledge described in the first sections of this chapter. In some senses this results in a conflation of lay and empirical knowledge to produce a model that is legitimised through both a scientific and popular discourse.

Popular epidemiology has at its roots the increasing concern with the environment as a cause of ill health, particularly in the context of pollution. Simple political protests against, for example, new roads, unsafe housing and polluted bathing water, formed the basis of the original movement. Popular epidemiology has carried these community protests further by hijacking the scientists' own domain of gathering and interpreting information. In other words this is epidemiological research by, and for the people.

Many examples of popular epidemiology exist in the USA, but a UK example, the pollution of the water supply in Camelford, will be discussed here. A more in-depth account may be found in Williams and Popay (1994a). The pollution occurred when 20 tonnes of aluminium sulphate was accidentally added to the water reservoir that supplied the residents of Camelford. A number of minor and major health problems, such as diarrhoea, headaches, fatigue and skin rashes were noted both by the population and by their medical practitioners. Following considerable local pressure a government enquiry led by Dame Barbara Clayton was convened. This reported that although the excess aluminium had had some immediate effects on health, delayed or persistent effects following such brief exposures were unlikely. The opposition of the local people to these conclusions was articulated through a support group and a scientific advisory panel of people who had academic and campaigning skills. This continuing collective and individual protest led to the reconvening of the Clayton Committee (with the same membership) to 'assess... persistent symptoms and clinicopathological findings amongst people who were resident in Camelford area at the time of the Lowermoor incident' (Department of Health, 1991b, p. 1). The committee reiterated the conclusions of the first enquiry.

At the heart of the dispute between the residents and the committee of enquiry was the claim to validity of the different types of evidence that both parties amassed. This was crystallised through a profound disjuncture between the perspectives of local people and experts concerning which type of evidence about the incident was 'admissible' (subjective and objective), and the mechanisms through which such data were interpreted. Both the first and second Clayton reports seem to imply that carefully collated information gleaned from people's own experience, because it represented subjective evidence, held little weight against the objective scientific evidence produced through toxicological and clinical measurements conducted under the auspices of the official inquiry. In opposition, the local residents refused to be disempowered by the authority of the scientists, claiming that their evidence was just as reliable as that of the committee. In doing this they directly challenged the epistemological basis of the epidemiological evidence produced by established science. Not only was this achieved by a refusal to accept that the evidence of the committee was impartial simply because it was produced through the scientific process, but also by their insistence that ethnographic data produced through the experience of local people could not be invalidated by reference to this same objective science (Williams and Popay, 1994a).

Developments such as those described above issue a challenge to the medicalisation of epidemiology through the precepts of lay knowledge. They are more than a political protest, for they represent a fundamental struggle over the meaning of health. Risks that are defined through the biomedical model as belonging to the individual are suddenly cast in a new light as public dangers. This of course represents a direct threat to mainstream epidemiology and the organisations associated with it. Popular epidemiology mobilises lay knowledge to critique the framework through which conventional epidemiology conceptualises and measures health risks (see also Chapter 6 for a further discussion of medical and lay conceptualisations of risk). From this evolves an emerging distrust of the experts who are doing the defining (Hayes, 1992), and a rebuttal of current public health policy.

If epidemiology continues to attempt to resolve the problems of public health solely through the epistemology of medicine its relevance to the real health problems of people will become obscured. A more pluralistic epidemiology which grasps perspectives emerging from different epistemologies and different players in the field of healthcare is what is required. This would challenge the notion that lay knowledge is the product of scientific ignorance and irrationality, and accept that such knowledge has equal legitimacy. Alongside this would need to be a commitment to broadening the range of methods through which research is conducted to include those qualitative designs that are commonly eschewed within science. If the new public health is truly a new enterprise, then the debate about health must be located in an 'ecological extension of democracy, where... a kind of "public science" would be charged as a second centre of the "discursive checking" of scientific laboratory results in the crossfire of opinions' (Beck, 1992a, p. 119). Once epidemiology is caught in this crossfire it will have to face up both to the limitations of its inherited medical model and to those health issues that are central to people's concern.

This chapter has attempted to lay bare some of the hidden (and not so hidden) assumptions that underlie orthodox epidemiology. The fundamental concepts of disease, illness, sickness and health have been examined from a variety of perspectives in order to analyse the various contributions that different disciplines bring to this field of enquiry. Nursing as an emerging discipline and a rapidly developing profession is in the enviable position of being able to more easily adopt and adapt such paradigms than either epidemiology itself or medicine. Chapter 6 will continue to expand on the debate started above, which is essentially centred on the polemic between positivism and naturalism. In particular, the routes through which nursing might pave the way to a more critical epidemiology will be discussed. This will be achieved through an exploration of specific examples, where the opportunities and constraints offered by epidemiology to nursing practice will be scrutinised. This more specific examination of practice must however, be situated in the wider context of the health service and nursing, which is explored in Chapters 3, 4 and 5.

CHAPTER THREE

Nursing, epidemiology and the National Health Service

It is not immediately apparent why a consideration of the organisation of nursing within the development of the health service should form part of a text on epidemiology. However, the milieu in which nurses work and act shapes the strategies that they adopt both in their clinical practice and in the research that they pursue. Nurses and nursing do not operate in a social vacuum. Individual professional practice and development is realised through an ongoing dynamic interaction, not only with other nurses, but also with many other professional and non-professional workers in the healthcare system.

Similarly, the structural and procedural regulations of organisations and professions will define the boundaries of individual and collective nursing action (Dingwall *et al.*, 1988). Such organisational limits may be overt, such as written procedures and policies, which cover particular issues, or they may act at a more subconscious level of 'cultural acceptance'. Thus certain practices are publicly identified and usually accepted and followed as the rules and regulations of the organisation, while others exist as part of the 'taken for granted' or accepted way of doing things at that time in that place.

These latter rules of living are certainly not written down, but form part of the tacit understandings which build up within any community. Every world has its own unique language and rituals which will alter subtly over time (Becker and Geer, 1970). Thus nurses speak of particular 'ward cultures' which encompass not only certain ways of working, but also an associated fund of stories and jokes which characterise that particular environment (Hardey, 1994). The ethos under which nurses work, and the people with whom they work, will thereby greatly influence any potential course of action or strategy that nursing might develop. Any reorganisation of health services, be it local or national, will perforce affect nursing to a greater or lesser extent depending on the nature and magnitude of the change. The almost continuous reorganisation of the National Health Service throughout the last two decades has had a profound effect on the professions integral to its function. A wider discussion of the social history of nursing may be found in Dingwall *et al.* (1988).

The first section of this chapter will examine the changes which have occurred and their implications for nursing. This contextualisation of nursing is necessary for a clearer understanding of how particular professional and research strategies may be constrained, or alternatively, unleashed by organisational boundaries. Thus the closer integration or uptake of epidemiology within nursing practice may be affected by such issues. For example, the history of the socio-political development of the professions within the health service, as outlined in this chapter, sheds light on why nursing has been reluctant to examine or adopt epidemiology, a discipline strongly associated with medicine, a profession to which nursing is historically subordinate.

THE NATIONAL HEALTH SERVICE

The National Health Service (NHS) began functioning on 5 July 1948 in accordance with the National Health Service Act of 1946. The NHS was explicitly based upon four principles – collectivism; comprehensiveness; universality; and equalitarianism (Allsop, 1984). Collectivism was reflected in the State's responsibility for its citizens, and hence for their health. Thus a service which was both comprehensive and free at the point of delivery was enshrined in the Act. The fragmented network of hospitals was in effect nationalised and finance was henceforth received through the Regional Hospital Boards, who were responsible to the Minister of Health. The provision of services was coordinated through the 14 regions of England and Wales. The service was devised to provide a complete but uniform range of healthcare to all citizens regardless of their wage-earning ability or place of residence.

Despite these changes, professional autonomy remained sacred in the new NHS. Bevan (1946) endorsed the central position of medicine thus: 'As I conceive it, the function of the Ministry of Health is to provide the medical profession with the best and most modern apparatus of medicine, and to enable them freely to use it, in accordance with their training for the benefit of the people of this country' (Allsop, 1984, p. 17).

This notwithstanding, two key devices effected control over the suppliers of a potentially uncertain healthcare system. The abolition of 'fee for service' restricted the extent of medical interventions to those that were strictly necessary, and the availability of consultant care only through GP referral controlled access to the most expensive 'areas' of the system, i.e. hospital care (Strong and Robinson, 1990). Nevertheless, clinical autonomy firmly placed decisions concerning expenditure and resource allocation in the province of consultants in hospitals and GPs in the community.

Medicine at this time has been described as the paradigmatic profession: 'a publicly mandated and state backed monopolistic supplier of a valued service, exercising autonomy in the workplace and collegiate control over recruitment, training and the regulation of members' conduct' (Elston, 1991, p. 58). This latter attribute of self-regulation is realised in syndicalism, which embodies the idea of independent practitioners whose professional conduct may not be questioned by outsiders. Syndicalism stamps its members with a common bond of long and arduous training, common practice and shared, but privileged, technical knowledge. It may thus act as an occupational power strategy. In one sense, then, the terms of the NHS provided for an emancipation from ill-informed external control (Honigsbaum, 1979), but from another perspective they were considered as the consolidation of medicine's monopolistic powers (Green, 1985a,b).

The syndicalist aspirations of British doctors were realised through the terms and conditions of their participation in the new health service. In turn, this meant that the NHS was not under the control of a manager, but 'the collective power of individual medical preference' (Strong and Robinson, 1990, p. 16). It was through this collective preference that nursing, despite its vastly superior numbers, remained subordinate to the medical endeavour. The development of the health service after 1948 was primarily focused on the delivery of medical care. This was a reflection both of official health policy and the dominant position of the medical profession in decision-making processes occurring both in hospitals and in the community. As Klein (1989, p. 54) puts it, during the 1950s 'the medical profession permeated the decision making machinery of the NHS at every level and achieved an effective right of veto over the policy agenda'.

THE RESTRUCTURING OF THE NHS AND NURSING

The workforce in the NHS has continued to increase in size. For example, by 1980 nurses represented 37% of NHS manpower and their numbers had doubled in the preceding decade (Office of Health Economics, 1982). This expansion in staff was coupled with an increasingly diverse division of labour within the health service professions. As a result, central government began to seek avenues for a more scientific management of the NHS. The first attempt was that of the Salmon Committee (Ministry of Health and Scottish Home and Health Department, 1966) which recommended that nursing services should be reorganised to create a tier of top and middle level managers separate from, and of higher rank to, practitioners and teachers. Although these changes were heavily criticised for engendering a culture where power and remuneration increased with distance from the patient (Carpenter, 1977), they did provide some preparation for the more effective participation of nursing in the changes of 1974.

The first major reorganisation of the NHS occurred in 1974 and involved the creation of district and area tiers of management, which were inserted between regions and hospitals. A new management ethos modelled on modern business lines was introduced, but essentially these changes remained bounded by the original framework of the NHS.

By this time hospital matrons had been replaced by Directors of Nursing Services, who now became subordinate to the District Nursing Officer. A new cadre of nurse administrators drawn from the ranks of practitioners was now firmly established. Two points need mentioning here. Firstly, nursing was ill equipped to undertake the financial and managerial responsibilities that were being thrust upon it. Yet the emerging clinical profession was additionally harnessed with the requirement for large numbers of skilled and professional managers. Secondly, as Strong and Robinson (1990, p. 18) observe, '1974 was... the apotheosis of health service syndicalism'. Each profession was to be managed, but managed separately by its own workers, coming together in consensus to manage the service as a whole (Department of Health and Social Security, 1972). However, consensus management, although creating the potential to plan and coordinate services, failed to address the fundamental divisions of power among the health service occupations, and underestimated their fierce tribalism. Encultured in a particularistic ethos, the professions were unable to take on board the more global perspectives necessary to providing a comprehensive and effective service. The reorganisation of 1974 was in essence an attempt to reconcile two conflicting policy aims: to increase managerial efficiency while continuing to placate the professions. In the event, no one was satisfied (Klein, 1989).

1984 saw a further reorganisation (DHSS, 1984) based upon the Griffiths inquiry (DHSS, 1983). Building on the 1982 changes, which introduced a layer of management at local or unit level, 'Griffiths' recommended a single leader or general manager for each tier. A management board for the NHS was set up, and for the first time a single line of command stretched from the top to the bottom of the service. The swift introduction of general managers heralded a more directive style. Charged with ensuring that resources were used efficiently and effectively, general managers 'cut a swathe across established lines of professional responsibility and clinical freedom' (Elston, 1991, p. 68). The then secretary of the RCN spelled out the implication of these changes 'The Griffiths inquiry... signalled the demise of professional power in the NHS. The doctors were deemed important only in so far as they could be nudged into management.... The nurses were deemed monumentally unimportant' (Clay, 1987, p. 57). Thus both medicine and nursing entered an era in which their professional power bases were inexorably eroded, and demands for managerial evaluation and control of clinical activities were increasingly heard (Maynard, 1988).

A more radical, and yet probably largely unplanned change, was on its way. In a television interview in 1988, Margaret Thatcher, facing a crisis in professional and public confidence in the NHS, announced that an internal government review of the service was under way. Seeking to encapsulate a further enhancement of efficiency and coordination within Mrs Thatcher's radical vision, the review group suggested a revolutionary solution – the internal market. Competition, absent from the NHS, might stimulate a cost-effective rise in input and quality of service; force clinicians to heed the cost of their activities; raise the profile of business principles in the service; and deflect problems away from the government towards the performance of local managers (Butler, 1992). The review body's white paper *Working for Patients* (Department of Health, 1989b) paved the way to the *Health of the Nation* (Department of Health, 1992a), which set targets for the reduction in coronary heart disease and stroke; cancers; mental illness; HIV/ AIDS and sexual health; and accidents. Thus for the first time not only were national objectives to achieving health set, but also the action and initiatives necessary to meet the targets, together with monitoring procedures, were established.

NURSING AND THE NHS IN THE 1990S

While the recent changes to the organisation of the NHS have spawned many criticisms, the realities are such that nurses and other healthcare professionals must continue to work within its confines. In this unpredictable and changing environment it is essential that nursing maximises the opportunities that reorganisation offers, while striving to deflect or change those aspects that detract from the equitable delivery of appropriate and humane care.

It is probably the 'market forces' component of the restructuring which causes most anguish to professionals weaned in a system where competition, business principles and, to an extent, costs were secondary considerations to the provision of a public service. The internal market has catapulted both providers and purchasers alike into a new culture of contested contracts and 'value for money' initiatives. Organisations, many of whom are now acting independently as hospital trusts, or GP fund-holders have responded by improving the efficiency, effectiveness and appropriateness of their services. In addition, the separation of providers and purchasers has made the choices of healthcare priorities, which existed covertly within the old system, more explicit and open to public scrutiny.

The framework of the new NHS is outlined in Figure 3.1 and the remainder of this section will consider the implications that these changes will have with particular reference to nursing and epidemiology.

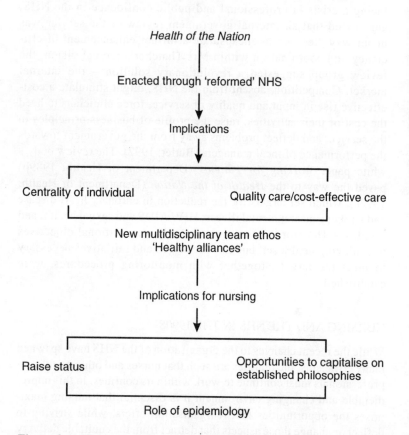

Figure 3.1 *The new NHS, nursing and epidemiology.*

Working through the new dynamic of the internal market, each profession must consider how it may best contribute to the restructured service. Certainly a momentum for change is apparent (Best *et al.*, 1994) and to a significant extent services are being reshaped (with or without consensual backing from the professions) to meet the targets set in *Health of the Nation*. Three other policy initiatives – *Caring for People* (Department of Health, 1989c), *The Children Act* (Department of Health, 1989d) and the *Patient's Charter* (Department of Health, 1991c) – will also have a major influence in shaping the form that nursing assumes over the next decade. A detailed account of the implications that these changes have for nursing and a framework through which nursing might act are contained in *A Vision for the Future* (Department of Health, 1993b) and *Testing the Vision* (Department of Health, 1994a). However, for the purposes of this book it is not so much the detail but the underlying changes in NHS culture which may inject new life into the neglected relationship between nursing and epidemiology.

The essence of the new NHS is contained in two principles: placing the users of the service and their carers at the centre of service provision, and a demand for quality care that is cost-effective (Figure 3.1). Running through much of the discourse is also the quest for a more open, equal and interactive relationship between the different professional groups, patients and their relatives. It is in this wider professional arena that nursing must make its mark. Indeed, if nursing 'keeps its head' the reorganisations may provide a framework on which the profession might capitalise. Two particular opportunities stand out – firstly, the possibility of raising the status of nursing as it is perceived by both other professionals and the public, and secondly the chance to bring to the forefront ideas such as holism and patient choice which have always ostensibly been part of nursing's philosophy, and which are now enshrined in the new legislation.

The dominance of biomedicine and the subservient position of nursing, although not openly acknowledged, are implicit in Duncan Nichol's foreword to *A Vision for the Future* (Department of Health, 1993b, p. iii): 'In order for... the nursing professions to achieve the targets... they will need the support of managers, doctors and other professional colleagues'. However, as Wright (Department of Health, 1993c) notes, Charter Statement no. 8, which states the requirement that each person should have a named, qualified nurse, midwife or health visitor 'is a public acknowledgement of the value of nursing'. This public statement of the worth of nursing not only raises the status of the profession, but also helps to dismiss the view of nursing as trivial women's work, highlighting instead the intricate and complex interpersonal and practical skills with which nursing is imbued. Thus a heightened sense of the societal worth of nursing has been engendered by the reforms, and this should enable the profession to form truly 'healthy alliances' where nurses stand in equal partnerships. In addition, the philosophy of nursing, its *modus operandi* and its practitioners have always been, and continue to be, in accord with the aims and objectives set out in *Caring for People* and *Health of the Nation*. In some senses, therefore, nursing has a head start in the struggle to refashion the nature of the services that are offered.

However, despite these advantages, it is clear that nursing, like the other professions, must be flexible and ready to adapt to new and imaginative ways of working in an alliance with rather different partners. With an increased focus on the health of local people, the reorganised service is very much concerned with efficiency, effectiveness and appropriateness of care. Much of the information necessary to underpin these new ways of working will be derived from epidemiology. For example, health authorities have been charged with assessing their population's need for healthcare and devising services and support which meet these needs (see Chapter 5). Much will be required in this area in terms of demographic and epidemiological survey research.

Similarly, the new emphasis on preventing illness and promoting health will incorporate many epidemiological strategies, such as screening, risk assessment and surveillance. In addition, health technology assessment, which encompasses 'the effectiveness, costs and broader impact of all procedures used by healthcare personnel to promote health and to prevent and treat illness' (Department of Health, 1992b, p. 16) is a government priority. Experimental epidemiological approaches, such as randomised controlled trials, will form the linchpin of many of the strategies to determine the relative merits of various clinical procedures and equipment.

Clearly, if nursing is to remain a major contender within the wider health service arena it is essential that it becomes familiar with the opportunities and constraints associated with the various epidemiological approaches that will be employed. It is crucial that nurses have a thorough grasp of the methodologies and principles behind these designs in order that they may utilise them effectively in their own work and evaluate their use by others. This expertise will be required not only by practitioners, but also by managers and educationalists. Whatever the setting, if nurses are competent to review critically the research pertaining to any proposed change in procedures or service, they will be confident to challenge and constructively add to the multidisciplinary debate.

The reorganised health service has placed much emp
provision of quality services to meet documented needs. It
ology that is increasingly providing the evidence for what
'quality' and what constitutes 'need'. It is thus within an
epidemiological paradigm that many of these questions a   ...ng
framed.

While epidemiology certainly has a prominent role to play in
moving forward the principles enshrined in the reorganisation, there
are many fundamental questions that require attention: for example,
what are health need and quality? A number of these issues will be
discussed at length in Chapter 5. However, this does not abrogate
nursing from the necessity to become familiar with epidemiology and
related subjects such as demography; rather, it makes the case more
strongly. It is these disciplines that will be extensively utilised both to
justify and to structure the initiatives associated with the reorganisations. Nursing and nurses must be able to both comprehend and
critique these developments from a sound knowledge base.

This chapter has thus far examined the historical and current position of nursing within a health service that has undergone both minor
and radical changes since its inception. This exploration has been
necessary to an understanding of the specific sociocultural milieu
which bounds nurses, their practice and their research. It has under-
lined the medical hegemony prevailing in the health service, and has
thus gone some way to explaining why nursing has striven to consoli-
date its own unique knowledge base and methods of research, different
from those of medicine. By examining the framework of the new NHS,
the possibilities, and indeed imperative challenges, that face nursing
as it nears the end of the century have been identified. The remainder
of the chapter will discuss how epidemiological designs might provide
the answers to some of these challenges. The reasons why these
designs have not been espoused so far by nursing will be the theme of
the final section.

THE CONTRIBUTION OF EPIDEMIOLOGY

Mainstream epidemiology has at its core a concern with delineating
the aetiology of acute and chronic conditions which affect humankind.
Through this central proposition it offers a set of techniques and a way
of thinking related to a determination of the natural history of a
condition; the factors that may contribute to that condition; and the
response of humans to those factors. This leads to the derivation of
strategies which may treat the condition or prevent it from appearing
or worsening. The central focus of the subject rests on the natural

history of conditions, including what does and does not occur before or after contact with healthcare professionals (some would define this latter process as the clinical course of the condition – see Chapter 1). This focus defines where epidemiological methods may be most useful. Traditionally, medicine has applied epidemiological methods for investigating a diverse set of activities, including (after Valenis, 1992):

- Determining the natural history of disease
- Identifying risk
- Classifying disease
- Diagnosing and treating disease
- Surveillance of health status
- Planning health services
- Evaluating health services

Determining the natural history of disease

The importance for epidemiology of the concept of the natural history of disease was discussed in Chapter 1. Knowledge of natural history is a necessary prerequisite to a thorough understanding of the aetiology and thus prevention of disease. In contrast with medicine, and to some extent nursing, epidemiology attempts to capture not only the later stages, where a condition becomes severe enough to require attention by the health service, but also the early pathogenic or prodromal stages, when either symptoms are ignored or people do not seek professional help. This provides a spectrum of disease severity that would not normally evolve through medical or nursing studies of patients under professional care. Information concerning the early natural history of conditions is essential to the planning of timely interventions or the identification and treatment of high-risk groups.

Identifying risk

When used in epidemiology, 'risk' refers to the probability that someone free of a condition, but who is exposed to certain risk factors, will subsequently acquire that condition.

Another related concept, which is sometimes confused with risk, is prognosis. Prognosis relates to the future course that a disease may take, and thus prognostic factors are conditions that may affect the outcome of those already known to have the disease. The outcome in risk factor studies is therefore a particular disease, whereas in studies of prognosis a variety of consequences of a disease are recorded. Risk factors are generally concerned with the prediction of low-probability events, whereas prognostic factors ascribe relatively frequent events. It is clear from this that although risk factors and prognostic factors may be the same, this is not necessarily so. For example, lack of exercise may be a risk factor for coronary heart disease, but it is not a prognostic factor determining outcome once a myocardial infarction has occurred.

Today's society is ever more aware of the risks surrounding it: risks in the environment (toxic waste, infectious agents); risks associated with sociocultural disruption (bereavement, war, famine); and inherited risks such as genetic disorders. Sometimes it is simple to recognise the relationship between exposure to a risk and an adverse outcome. Such is the case with many infectious diseases. However, for chronic diseases of multiple aetiology the relationship between risks and disease is less clear. In these cases it is difficult for clinicians to develop estimates of risk based on their own limited experience. Some of the reasons for this include long latency; frequent exposure to risk factors; low incidence of disease; and multiple causes and effects (Fletcher *et al.*, 1988). All these situations may contrive to ensure that an individual practitioner perhaps will not see the resulting outcome following an exposure, ever see a case of the condition in question, or see enough patients to determine which of many possible risk factors are the most important. Both risk and prognosis may be determined using cohort studies (see Chapter 1). The identification of risks allows the construction of screening programmes and health promotion strategies aimed at changing high-risk behaviours. This is a particularly important area for nursing, which will be more fully discussed in Chapter 6.

Classifying disease

Epidemiological data allows the identification of clusters of signs and symptoms as particular disease entities. This classification system is the linchpin of modern biomedicine, and it allows the matching of individual symptoms with published case definitions (The International Classification of Diseases). However, although this tactic is undoubtedly useful in epidemiological terms, the scientific classification of diseases may cause more problems than it solves. For example, definitions of psychiatric disease applied cross-culturally have been condemned as meaningless and even harmful (Kleinman, 1987; Lewis *et al.*, 1990). Given the marked variation between what is considered 'normal' in different parts of the world, can mental illness in different societies be assigned the same labels (Helman, 1990)? The problems associated with disease and disease classifications are discussed more fully in Chapter 2.

Disease

		Present	Absent	
Result of screening test	Positive	a	b	a+b
	Negative	c	d	c+d
		a+c	b+d	a+b+c+d

Sensitivity = $a / (a + c)$
Specificity = $d / (b + d)$
Positive predictive value = $a / (a + b)$
Negative predictive value = $d / (c + d)$
Prevalence = $(a + c) / (a + b + c + d)$

Figure 3.2 *Specifications for screening or diagnostic tests*

Diagnosing and treating disease

A major proportion of doctors' time is occupied with determining a diagnosis for any individual patient who consults them. This activity includes ruling out other diagnoses, and often involves the application of diagnostic tests. The interpretation of these tests is not quite as straightforward as it might appear. There are certain mathematical relationships between the properties of tests (such as their sensitivity and specificity[1]) and the information that they produce in different clinical situations. Test results may present four possible scenarios, as depicted in Figure 3.2. Two are correct – a positive test in the presence of disease and a negative test in the absence of disease.

However, tests may mislead clinicians when they present false positive (i.e. a positive test with no disease) or false negative (i.e. a negative test when disease is present) results. The implications of such false results depend rather on the condition in question. For example, it would not be too serious if a false positive test of a mid-stream urine sample indicated that a patient had an infection and should be treated with antibiotics. On the other hand, if a patient with cervical cancer was given a false negative result, the disease might progress beyond a

---

1   **Sensitivity** is defined as the proportion of people who have disease and who have a positive test for that disease. A very sensitive test will seldom miss people with the disease in question. **Specificity** is defined as the proportion of people without the disease who test negative. A very specific test will therefore rarely misclassify undiseased people into the diseased category.

stage amenable to treatment. New diagnostic tests are usually compared with a 'gold standard' (the best possible assessment of whether disease is present or not – perhaps an expensive radiological technique or autopsy results) to determine their appropriateness for use in different situations. A very clear and concise description of diagnostic tests and their application may be found in Fletcher *et al.* (1988).

Surveillance and planning and evaluating of health services

Surveillance is defined as close observation or invigilation. In epidemiology it involves the collection of relevant data, analysis and interpretation of those data, and finally the dissemination of the information that has been found. Surveillance data provide information about who is most at risk of contracting a disease and where and when diseases are most frequently observed. This information will be useful not only in the early detection of problems, but also for the strategic planning of healthcare services. Monitoring conditions in this way can alert health professionals to trends or unusual clusters of events. In Britain, many infectious diseases, such as diphtheria, tuberculosis and anthrax, must be notified to the appropriate authorities within 48 hours of their diagnosis. In this way outbreaks may be identified and hopefully confined. Surveillance of other conditions, such as birth defects, may point to the possible involvement of causal agents. The role of epidemiology in providing information and statistics which are used for planning services is examined more closely in Chapters 4 and 5, whilst Chapter 6 provides a specific example of the use of surveillance in nursing.

By providing information and statistics about the community's health, epidemiology allows the nature and size of different problems to be assessed objectively. Knowledge about the distribution of disease according to geographical location, age, ethnic origin, socio-economic group etc. is necessary for planning the extent and types of services that are required by any particular population. Indeed, an overriding theme of *Working for Patients* (Department of Health, 1989b) and many of the subsequent proposals produced by regional health authorities was the necessity for determining the health needs of communities (Department of Health, 1993d). Epidemiology can certainly provide the tools for such analyses, but the caveats in the next chapter concerning the origins and reliability of healthcare information should be carefully noted. Such data are not produced in a moral and social vacuum, and just as epidemiological studies may be prone to statistical bias, so may the gathering and interpretation of statistics be open to 'socio-political bias'.

EPIDEMIOLOGY IN NURSING

This section has so far expanded on the medical uses of epidemiology, but nursing may also need to use some of these approaches, perhaps in a modified format, and albeit in a framework of care different from that of medicine. Chapters 1 and 2 discussed some of the limitations to traditional epidemiology, particularly those related to its foundation within 'science'. Nursing has already adopted a more flexible and holistic model of health and illness, and might thus be in a strong position to champion some of the newer developments in social and lay epidemiology. As Williams and Popay (1994b, p. 104) suggest 'Many health problems... require more flexible definitions of research, science and data'. Many nurses working in several different arenas, for example community care, school health, rehabilitation, infection control and occupational health, have had cause to use epidemiological methods in their research or everyday work (Cook, 1981). This use of epidemiology in nursing frequently mirrors its use in medicine and follows closely along the lines described in the section above. Epidemiology may be of special value to nursing in three instances:

- where it enhances approaches already adopted (such as in the design of quantitative research)
- where it fulfils a pressing need within nursing (such as in the critical review of the literature)
- where its uptake by nursing poses some fundamental questions concerning the discipline of epidemiology itself (such as the validity of current biomedical disease classification systems)

These theoretical opportunities crystallise into five main areas where nursing might take most benefit from the epidemiological approach as:

- a model for quantitative nursing research
- a strategy for evaluating the clinical nursing research literature
- a framework for thinking for clinical decisions
- a mechanism for the effective and efficient planning and delivery of nursing services *to those who most need them*
- an opportunity to enrich current nursing concepts, or to create new and mutually enhancing shared theory.

As a **model for quantitative research**, epidemiology offers an array of designs, such as cohort studies, prevalence surveys and randomised controlled trials, which facilitate the objective study of healthcare phenomena and practices. The meticulous control measures that epidemiology has recognised and implemented in observational studies have allowed the rigorous study of real-life situations, which under normal circumstances would not be amenable to experimental investigations (see Chapter 1). Where nurse researchers do adopt quantitative methodologies epidemiology often provides a tried and tested framework through which studies may be planned.

Although utilising an epidemiological methodology in their studies, many nurse researchers do not allude to this in their reports. Indeed it is possible that some of them are unaware that they have adopted an epidemiological stance. Since not only nurses, but also many biological and social scientists who may be engaged in nursing research, lack specific training in epidemiology, this is not surprising. Although examples of most types of epidemiological design may be found in the nursing literature, cohort studies have been particularly favoured (Jacobsen and Meininger, 1985). Some examples include a prospective study of women's roles and illness episodes (Woods, 1980); Cullum and Clark's investigation of the intrinsic factors associated with the development of pressure sores in elderly people (1992); and research by Ballard and McNamara (1983) to determine nursing needs in home healthcare. These studies exemplify some of the medical uses of epidemiology (for example, the identification of risk factors and the planning of healthcare services), but situate their use within nursing.

The Briggs Report of 1972 catalysed the effort to establish nursing as a research-based profession. However, although numerous documents and papers since then (Department of Health 1989a, 1993a; MacFarlane 1984) have reiterated this call, the mechanisms by which this research grounding is to be achieved are seldom clarified (Hardey and Mulhall, 1994). However, a fundamental requisite is that at least some, if not all, nurses should acquire an ability to **critically evaluate the research literature**. Until recently, nursing education did not provide students with the depth of methodological understanding that would enable them to undertake or even appreciate research, and some disciplines, such as sociology, have only found a place in the nursing curricula since 1970 (Perry, 1987).

The new Project 2000 courses and the move towards integration with higher education should inject a much-needed boost to the effort to develop a research culture within nursing. These changes should ensure that more practitioners are able to understand and critically assess research than at present (Armitage, 1990; Millar, 1993). The acquisition of 'research awareness' or 'research literacy' does not imply that all practitioners should undertake research. Rather, it strives to produce a climate in which research reports are sought out, critically reviewed, and their potential for practice recognised.

One obstacle to achieving this goal is the sheer volume of reports produced and their inconsistent quality. The literature related to healthcare is expanding by 6–7% each year (de Solla Price, 1981). The time available to any individual to obtain and read such material is also diminishing. All articles are not of equal importance, and it is necessary to seek out the most valid, reliable and appropriate studies from the great mass produced. Improvements in the care of patients will only occur where rigorous research has been used as the basis for new initiatives. Epidemiology offers a set of strategies for reading and organising the literature, in particular quantitative studies, in a systematic way. The critical assessment of research reports is integral to modern nursing. Not only must practitioners be proficient appraisers of such material, but managers and purchasers or commissioners of health services must also be able to recognise significant research findings. The importance of this subject and its critical bearing on the establishment of nursing as a credible profession merits its more detailed examination in Chapter 7.

Clinical decision-making is integral to many of the activities subsumed under nursing's umbrella of providing care or medicine's rubric of cure. While ostensibly centred on the diagnostic process, decision-making occurs throughout other processes (Hunter, 1980). For most of us, most of the time, decisions seem to occur automatically and any 'processing' is rarely brought into consciousness . At other times, specific problems occur which force us to wrestle with a variety of choices with, or without the benefit of relevant information.

Are different processes involved in taking these decisions? In practice are there different sort of decisions and are they accorded different approaches to their solution? These are questions which must be left to psychology to answer (Llewelyn and Hopkins, 1993). Medical epidemiology has taken another approach based on quantitative decision-making. Decision analysis in a clinical context may be defined as 'a method of describing complex clinical problems in an explicit fashion, identifying the available courses of action... assessing the probability and value of all possible outcomes, and then making a simple calculation to select the optimal course of action (Sackett *et al.*, 1991, p. 139). This then is the mathematical modelling of clinical problems. It provides one legitimate avenue to answering the sort of questions that face all nurses in their daily practice. This strategy is explained in detail, and some cautionary notes to its use provided in Ransohoff and Feinstein (1976) and Weinstein *et al.* (1980).

This book is concerned at a more general level with the ways in which information is collected and interpreted than in these other approaches to decision-making. As individual nurses encounter old or fresh presentations of sickness, their courses of action will be influenced by numerous factors. How much do they know from theory or experience about the situations they face? Are there specific organisational or professional guidelines that must be followed? In what ways is the encounter affected by the sociocultural milieu in which it is occurring? Does the research literature offer any information on the subject? Nurses are attempting to particularise to the individual their experiences with other similar patients.

Clinical epidemiology attempts to provide a scientific basis for clinical observations. It provides a method of assessing the validity of the clinical judgements that nurses make in their everyday practice. Maximising the efficiency and effectiveness of healthcare, and perforce the judgements relating to it, is the central theme underlying much of the recent restructuring of the UK health service. Whether this will result in a more equitable, accessible and acceptable service is questionable, but nurses and their medical colleagues must function within the new system. Indeed, at face value there is nothing to lose and everything to gain by attempting to determine *the most effective strategies for managing and providing nursing services to those who most need them*. Epidemiology provides the framework whereby effective strategies are identified.

In May 1991, the Director of Research and Development for the NHS convened an advisory group to consider methods for assessing the effects of health technologies. Their report adopted a broad view on the term 'health technologies' to include 'the variety of methods used by health professionals to promote health, to prevent and treat disease, and to foster improved rehabilitation and long term care' (Department of Health 1992b, p. 4). The methods therefore embraced 'hardware', such as equipment and medicines, and 'software', such as diagnostic and therapeutic policies, skills and people's time. Health technology assessment under these terms covers a multitude of activities in which nurses, doctors and other professional healthcare workers are involved.

A word of caution is perhaps timely here. Nursing has firmly embraced 'care' as central to its enterprise, but the definition of care and its epistemological status are problematic (Thomas, 1993). Difficulties may therefore be encountered in convincing a sceptical medical hegemony that such a concept can stand up to scientific scrutiny. Under these inauspicious circumstances, studies of nursing care may fall by the wayside. Although the prescription of drugs is largely outwith nursing's remit, nurses both within and outside institutional settings have frequently to select and monitor equipment provided to their patients. Hundreds of items, such as urinary catheters, walking aids and pressure-relieving mattresses, are used each day. However, again the items that nurses use are frequently at the 'mundane' end of the spectrum, and suggestions that their effectiveness should be tested may meet with little enthusiasm.

Despite these cautions it is obvious that health technology assessment will play a major role in nursing research and development. Nursing needs to be aware of the potential that epidemiology has for providing the framework through which such assessments may be made, and Chapter 6 explores this area more fully. Some practices will be more amenable than others to conventional epidemiological evaluation. Where an intervention or a strategy for care may be closely defined and its outcome easily ascertained by reliable and valid measures, the quantitative methods of epidemiology will find a use.

Another major aspect of nursing concerns the early recognition of impending ill health. This forms the rationale for any type of routine or selective screening programme. A second strand to this activity revolves around the surveillance of populations and the assessment of factors that may enhance or decrease any individual's chance of becoming sick. Connected to this is the recent trend towards promoting health rather than merely detecting disease when it appears. As with diagnostic tests, screening tests may be subjected to epidemiological scrutiny and, as discussed above, estimating risk and surveillance also fall within the remit of epidemiology. It is just as important to be aware of the limitations of a screening test as it is to understand the efficiency of a particular treatment.

In some senses the screening and surveillance of the 'normal' population carries additional burdens of responsibility. Healthy people are just that: they have constructed and continue to construct their everyday lives on this basis. Informing them that they may be carriers of a certain disease, or have a propensity to develop a certain condition may have an irreversible and detrimental effect on their entire lives. If no suitable treatment is available, or where the value of the diagnostic indicator is questionable, then uncomfortable questions need to be posed as to the value of screening in the first place. Before any screening programme is implemented, careful consideration must be given to the ethical aspects that may arise. These topics – screening, prevention, surveillance and assessment of risk are important both to nursing and to epidemiology, and they will be further explored in Chapter 6.

Constraints to using epidemiology in nursing

In their desire to establish the credibility of nursing research, early workers espoused objective scientific methodologies modelled on those used in biomedicine (Abdellah and Levine, 1971; Polit and Hungler, 1983). However, the last fifteen years have witnessed a growing polemicism between these researchers and others who consider that the social world can be investigated only through more qualitative methodologies, such as phenomenology, which strives to capture the lived experience of those who it studies (Duffy, 1985).

As discussed in Chapter 1 this disavowal of quantitative research is a crystallisation of a number of factors, both ideological and structural, which conspire to enhance the position of the qualitative stance. The ideology of nursing is not one of 'hard objective science': both the public's view and the profession's own view of itself are bound up in notions of care. Founded on an uneasy partnership between Christian duty and emotional love, care is a Janian domain – ostensibly prized, and yet devalued by society as mere 'women's work'. Although 'high-tech' nursing, such as that which occurs in intensive care units, may be perceived by the public as scientific, the majority of nursing care is not constructed in this framework, either by the public or a large part of the profession (Dunlop, 1986).

How, many nurses might ask, can epidemiology contribute to a paradigm of nursing which embraces these concepts? Many organisational structures also inhibit any appreciation or adoption of epidemiological techniques by nurses. There is an acute shortage of lecturers in nursing departments who are capable of teaching more than the rudiments of epidemiology. Few nursing courses thus include epidemiology in their curricula, and where they do it is the traditional mainstream branch of the discipline that is taught. Exploration of aspects of social epidemiology or the New Public Health (Ashton and Seymour, 1991) receives little attention. In addition, epidemiology and demography demand an appreciation of statistics, in which many nurses are either ill prepared, or embedded from an early stage into a culture of 'number aversion'.

Not only is there a lack of formal teaching of epidemiology, but there is also a dearth of nursing research within this area. This, not unnaturally, is related to the scarcity of lecturing staff possessing a thorough training in epidemiology. Staff in institutes of higher education often act as role models for future career aspirations, and students' research projects frequently form the springboard for subsequent more ambitious pieces of research. Where epidemiology receives little recognition, where there are no nurse researchers active in the area and where only a small proportion of the curriculum is devoted to this subject, it is hardly surprising that epidemiology is not espoused more widely. The constraints to using epidemiology in nursing are therefore based both in concrete organisational structures, such as nurse education, and in more ephemeral ideas concerning nursing as 'soft work' or 'women's work', which do not stand up to hard scientific scrutiny.

The hierarchical nature of healthcare work and the consequent divisions between both the professional and non-professional staff engaged in such work are well recognised (Stacey, 1988). Epidemiology has traditionally been situated firmly within medicine, and thus many nurses may consign its methods to a domain in which they do not consider playing (indeed, they do not wish to play) a part. This intellectual process of automatically equating epidemiological methods or processes with the parent discipline, which is itself redolent of medicine, may thereby deprive nursing of a rich source of rigorous methodologies. Ironically epidemiology itself has endured an equally low status when compared with clinical medicine (Levine and Lilienfeld, 1987). This is partly a reflection of epidemiology's association with the public health profession, whose prestige within the medical hierarchies is equally low. Western medicine reserves the highest plaudits for pursuits that embrace high technology and the expertise associated with it (Daniels, 1971). As Levine and Lilienfeld (1987, p. 4) note: 'despite their enormous implications for health, getting people to stop smoking or wear seat belts... – all appear unglamorous pursuits compared to transplanting organs...'. Nursing has a remarkably similar legacy of recognition by today's society.

Historically, nurses have participated in research studies that were led by professionals from another discipline, for example sociology or medicine. The preponderance of vacancies for 'Nurse Researchers' at low (F or G) staffing grades advertised in the press is testimony to the junior position that nurses often occupy in such research teams. This creates two problems. Firstly, nurses employed for these projects are frequently assigned to collect data (usually quantitative) using instruments that have already been chosen and designed by other members of the team. Their involvement in other aspects of the research may be slight and the opportunity to learn how to conduct research themselves may thereby be lost. These posts are therefore often perceived *post hoc* as unfulfilling, and they further the division between nursing and the other professions involved in healthcare research.

Secondly, the preponderance of positions at these lower grades subsumes a tacit assumption by others that nurses are only capable of participation in the more routine aspects of research. The social construction of a research world in which nursing is both marginal and subordinate is implicit in these employment strategies. In addition, an erroneous image of nursing research as being principally concerned with data collection by relatively junior personnel is perpetuated. By devaluing the individual and collective experience of research, this image may influence the manner in which many practising nurses view the wider research enterprise. These problems are not only confined to the subjugation of nursing research. Where professionals other than nurses are leading a project the content and framing of the questions asked, although valuable in their own right, may not address the concerns of nursing or the people they seek to help. The contextualisation of nursing research within the wider research world may therefore conspire towards either an ignorance, or a dismissal, of epidemiological approaches by nurses. How this trend may be reversed, leading to a more open, yet critical espousal of epidemiology within nursing, will be explored through a number of specific examples in Chapter 6.

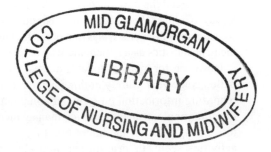

CHAPTER FOUR

Health information and statistics

The primary focus of epidemiology is the distribution of disease in the population and the factors that affect this. The measurement of disease frequency and the determination of its complex relationship with demographic characteristics is therefore a central activity. Good information concerning the health status of communities and the trends prevailing over time has always been central to epidemiology, and the key to public health. Indeed the importance of health statistics forms part of nursing's legacy (Cohen, 1984), for it was Nightingale who, working with the statistician William Farr, was one of the first to recognise the potential of medical statistics as a systematic way of learning from experience.

However, for many of today's nurses, the attraction of statistics has palled somewhat. Surely nothing can be more irksome than tediously recording information on forms or computers only to see it disappear into the jungle of health service management. Many nurses and doctors strongly resent the hours that they are forced to devote to such activities, seeing them as time spent 'away from the client'. As a result, discussions of population statistics and trends generate little enthusiasm among practitioners. In addition, the generally poor level of statistical competence among healthcare professionals militates against their participation in such discussions at an informed level.

Furthermore, nursing in particular has taken as its focus the individual, and extending this ideology to encompass groups of individuals or populations may be troublesome. For practitioners, whose major commitment and workload revolves around one-to-one interactions with clients, the significance of statistics about the wider community may not be readily apparent.

This chapter cannot hope to radically alter these attitudes to health statistics. It does, however, aim to provide a clear description of how such statistics are compiled, some of the problems associated with their collection, and the possible uses to which they are put.

All health information data needs to be collected consistently and recorded accurately to be of maximum benefit. The reorganisation of the NHS has resulted in an increasing emphasis on such 'hard' data both as a source of information for planning healthcare services and as a benchmark for undertaking monitoring activities like quality assurance and audit, in which nursing is involved. Epidemiology and demography form the foundation through which health statistics are collected, analysed and presented, and an appreciation of these processes will enable nursing to participate fully in issues more usually reserved for the domain of public health.

The recording and compilation of health statistics is a complex and intricate task. This chapter will describe the different types of measure used to describe health and disease and how they are calculated. It will also give some indications as to the mechanisms through which the reliability and accuracy of data may be assessed. Being faced with a set of well-presented statistical tables and graphs calls for some epidemiological resources in order that such information may be objectively evaluated. Which population exactly do these data represent? What information is missing? How have categories been constructed? Who collected the data? Why were the data collected? These are the types of question that an informed nurse epidemiologist will ask.

Furthermore, statistical information about the public 'health' is no more immune from the social and politico-economic environment than the many other epidemiological issues covered in this book. Statistics are usually portrayed as a technical discipline unaffected by social values or ideology. This portrayal is misleading: just because knowledge has been produced in a numerical format does not automatically guarantee that it is objective. Proponents of non-neutrality contend that statistical data are 'socially produced in specific circumstances (for example under the auspices of a funding agency and a research unit), for specific reasons (government use in planning social programs...) and with techniques developed and transformed in historically specific ways' (Turshen, 1989, p. 42 after Irvine *et al.*, 1979). The social and political dimensions of data and their collection, analysis and presentation (or suppression) are themes which will be explored in the final section.

Perhaps it is apposite to end this introduction with two quotes. One is derived from the transcripts of a seminar held in 1974 at the London School of Hygiene and Tropical Medicine to examine the future of government health statistics. The final discussion makes the comment that 'simple statistics conceal more than they reveal and... that the provision, interpretation, and use of data are extremely complex and contentious matters' (Acheson *et al.*, 1976, p. 131). The second quote comes from Bailar (1976, p. 117) who suggests that 'there may be greater danger to the public welfare from statistical dishonesty than from almost any other form of dishonesty'.

TYPES AND SOURCES OF HEALTH STATISTICS

Much of the information about health statistics is derived through the work of demographers. Demography is the study of whole populations and the trends that such populations undergo over time.

Some of the questions that demographers might pose are: how many births occur in a certain geographical area? What is the age profile of a particular population? Is the proportion of people over the age of 65 years increasing or decreasing? Not only does demography record these statistics, but it also attempts to predict how they will change over time. It is this type of demographic data that epidemiologists frequently use as the basis for their work.

Health statistics may be collected as part of a discrete exercise or research project: for example, many surveys have been conducted recently in particular hospitals or district health authorities to determine the prevalence of pressure sores (Nyquist and Hawthorn, 1987; Dealey, 1991). Of more importance to epidemiology are the statistics that are collected routinely through various health authority and government agencies. The three principal types of routinely collected information are population data, mortality data and morbidity data.

Population data

The census, which is coordinated by the Office of Population Censuses and Surveys (OPCS), is the single most important source of information concerning the size and composition of the population. A census has occurred in Great Britain every 10 years since 1801, with the exception of 1941. Population estimates that take account of births, deaths and migration are also made for the years in-between censuses. Also undertaken are long-term forecasts, or population projections, which attempt to estimate future trends based on information from the last census. The size and structure of future populations in this case has to be based on assumptions about future migration, mortality and fertility rates. The last of these rates has, through past experience proved extremely difficult to forecast, leading to grossly inaccurate predictions of population projections. In the short term (perhaps 20 years), however, such predictions may be relatively accurate.

Population projections have a multitude of uses, but in the area of health they are used in the strategic planning of future services that will be sufficient and appropriate to a population's needs. The census thus provides reliable data on the size and structure of the population, which enables planners to determine the nature and extent of the health services required in any area. In addition, these data are used to estimate the size of the population 'at risk' of any condition, and this provides the denominator for calculating rates (see the next section). For example, fertility rates cannot be calculated without a knowledge of how many women of childbearing age exist in a community: in an area which has a high proportion of retired people living in it, the rate of births per woman might be low, although the actual fertility rate for childbearing women might be similar to other regions.

There are some problems associated with the population data obtained through the census. The reliability and accuracy of the data obtained through this source depend not only on the data collection process, but also on the people filling in the forms. Some of these difficulties relate to conscious decisions that individuals make in completing or not completing their returns, and others to genuine misunderstandings or administrative problems, for despite completion being compulsory by law some under-reportage may occur. Although the census aims to enumerate all the population, it never achieves this target. Particular sources of under-coverage include very young children and the homeless. In addition, certain items of information, such as age or occupation, may be distorted or too vague (in the latter case) for an accurate return to be made. This may have important consequences, for occupation is used as the basis for determination of social class, a variable upon which much future epidemiological research may be based.

As noted above, long-term population forecasts may be grossly distorted by our inability to accurately predict future fertility rates, and current population estimates may be distorted by the patchy information which is available concerning internal migrations. In this latter case substantial errors in population statistics for small areas may occur.

Mortality data

The notification of deaths in Great Britain began in 1532, and the first attempts at a nationwide registration of vital events commenced in 1538. However, compulsory registration of births, deaths and marriages occurred even earlier (AD 720) in Japan.

Most Western countries now have a relatively accurate and reliable system for generating mortality statistics. For example, in the UK a Registrar's Certificate or Coroner's Order is required for disposal of a body. This legal requirement, linked with the nature of an event which is rarely in doubt, gives mortality data an edge over other health statistics. The occurrence of death is therefore usually accurately and reliably recorded, but another factor which is of paramount interest in many epidemiological studies is the cause of death. In Great Britain the physician who attended the deceased in his or her last illness is required by law to complete a medical certificate of death on which the cause of death must be stated. This certificate is then taken by a qualified informant (usually the closest relative of the deceased) to the local Registrar of Deaths. Here other details including the date and place of death, name, sex, date and place of birth, occupation and place of residence of the deceased are provided orally by the informant. At weekly intervals the registrar then makes a death return to OPCS where the information on the certificates is coded. For most of the information this is straightforward, but coding for the cause of death is more complex (see below).

The comprehensiveness, easy availability and reliability of mortality statistics has historically ensured them a place in many epidemiological studies. Routine mortality statistics are published annually by many countries, and the World Health Organisation produces regular information concerning the population demographics and mortality rates of as many countries as possible. Mortality statistics are also particularly useful in the study of occupational factors that might lead to increased rates of death. A difficulty here however, is that although the numerator for such mortality rates is known from the records at OPCS, the denominator, i.e. the number of people pursuing this occupation, is only known accurately (or relatively accurately) at the time of each 10-year census.

Again, an early example of the use of occupational mortality data is provided by William Farr, who analysed the mortality rate by cause of hospital employees. Nightingale, in her *Notes on Hospitals* (1863), records Farr's results, which indicated that the annual mortality from contagious diseases was more common in matrons, sisters and nurses than in the 'female population of London'.

Although mortality data are useful there is an increasing redundancy in their use, since most important diseases, in the Western world at least, are chronic, remitting and of long duration. In this situation mortality data cannot adequately describe the 'health' (or 'disease') of a population. Historically, when acute infectious diseases were more important, mortality rates provided a much more accurate reflection of the relative frequency and distribution of particular diseases, since people either died quickly of the affliction or were cured. Under these conditions mortality rates are a reliable monitor of the health of a population. The decline in importance of acute infectious diseases as a cause of death in the 20th century has led to the development of other systems of information to collect statistics on illness or morbidity in the community. Some of these will be discussed in the next section.

The official nature of the events surrounding the recording of deaths and the perceived status of the governmental bodies dealing with such matters may lull the unwary user of such statistics into a false sense of security. There is no doubt that mortality statistics are both comprehensive and reliable, at least in Western countries, but such data must be viewed critically. There are several points in the system where errors may occur.

Firstly, mistakes may be made in the recording of the cause of death. Several studies in the UK and USA have demonstrated that the cause on the certificate may differ from the cause related in the person's medical notes or the cause as revealed by post-mortem examination. In addition, the cause of death as ascertained by the doctor is based purely on clinical opinion, as post-mortem examination only occurs in a minority of cases. Discrepancies are more likely in the elderly, where the precise cause of death may be unclear or several multiple causes may be responsible. In a younger person more thorough investigation of the cause of death is likely to occur.

Once the data is in the hands of the OPCS coders, further difficulties may arise. Coders at the OPCS use the International Classification of Diseases issued by the World Health Organisation to translate the underlying cause of death, i.e. the 'morbid condition which started the chain of events' into a code. However, there are occasions when the diagnosis is vague, or an illogical sequence of events is presented, and in these cases the coders resort to a predetermined set of rules to try to disentangle the problem. It is clear that errors can occur at this stage. In addition, as Donaldson and Donaldson (1993, p. 23) note, 'it seems increasingly illogical to cling to the notion of a single underlying morbid process, hence experiments are under way to explore multi-cause coding of death'.

A second area where discrepancies may occur is in the provision of information by the qualified informant. In practice this informant is usually the deceased's closest relative. Since deaths must be registered within five days of their occurrence, this person is probably in a highly emotional state and likely to provide confused or inaccurate information. In particular, serious errors relating to the reporting of occupation may occur. The qualified informant, even if he or she is the spouse, may not know exactly what the deceased did, or may consciously or unconsciously elevate the deceased's position. Also, the deceased person's last occupation may well not have been what the majority of his or her life was spent doing. These potential discrepancies are important because occupation is used to determine social class. Inaccuracies may therefore distort the reported differential risk of death amongst the different social classes. In addition, information relating mortality to occupation may identify certain workers who are more at risk of dying from certain causes. This may highlight occupational exposures that are putting particular groups of workers at risk of certain diseases.

Even with an event as discrete and definite as death, therefore, some limitations on the accuracy and reliability of the data will be imposed through the method of collection and the prevailing laws and customs of the society in which the information is compiled. Nevertheless, mortality data, because of their accessibility and relative completeness, are often used as the first step in defining a health problem. However, the demise of many acute and fatal conditions to history has instigated the development of other indices through which the health of populations may be described. These are the statistics on morbidity.

Morbidity data

Data describing morbidity provide information about sickness in communities, whether or not this sickness results in death. Again, OPCS is responsible in England and Wales for the collection and presentation of these data on a national basis. Several diverse types of morbidity data have been collected routinely from different population groups. These include information on hospital in-patients (1949–85); patients attending GPs (1955–56, 1970–71, 1981–82); and 'the general population' in the General Household Survey (every year since 1971). In addition, statistics are collected routinely on abortions, congenital malformations, cancers, infectious diseases, incapacity to work, adverse drug effects, sickness absence and industrial accidents.

Two crucial characteristics define much of the morbidity data collected. Firstly, they are usually based on the use of NHS facilities, and secondly they often rely on notification from individual practitioners.

In 1982 the Steering Group on Health Services Information (the Körner Committee) reviewed the main sources of morbidity data available from hospitals. These included the Hospital Activity Analysis (HAA), which recorded demographic, clinical and administrative data for every episode of in patient care; the Hospital Inpatient Enquiry (HIPE), which was made obligatory in 1957 and involved the statistical analysis of a 10% sample of data from HAA; the annual hospital returns, which provided data by speciality for number of available beds, number of discharges, average length of stay and waiting lists; and the Mental Health Enquiry, which provided similar data on mental health patients.

The data collected by these information systems are clearly limited. Some of these limitations relate to the methods of collecting and recording information. For example, HAA and HIPE only record data on each episode of care, unrelated to the individual. In other words, the system counts events and not people, and thus a monthly discharge rate of 20 for diabetes might include 20 people with diabetes or 10 people who had each entered hospital twice because of their diabetic condition. In addition, the accuracy of the clinical data included in HAA is severely limited by the failure of many clinicians to provide the relevant information, which through default must be derived from the patients' notes by the coding clerk in the medical records department. This provides a salient insight into the value that practitioners place on health statistics.

Another limitation of hospital morbidity data is that by definition it only relates to people who actually become in-patients. The ability of these indices to measure accurately the extent of disease morbidity in any given population is therefore confined (a) to those people who consult a medical practitioner and enter hospital, and (b) to those conditions that merit entry to hospital. Many prevalent and/or serious diseases do not fall into these categories.

The national morbidity studies of general practice aimed to capture some of the information that is inevitably omitted from hospital morbidity data. Following the establishment of an age/sex register, the participating GPs recorded information such as diagnosis, dates of consultation and any subsequent referrals on each 'sickness episode'. These surveys probably represent the best available data on less serious sickness (at least as defined within a biomedical paradigm), but there are limitations. As with the hospital data, the catchment of information relies on the patient entering the health service system. The GPs who participated were self-selected and not a random sample, and thus the data produced may be biased. Finally, in the long term there is no existing mechanism through which the scheme could be extended to all GPs, and indeed there are no financial incentives for them to undertake such work.

Health statistics derived from self-assessment, such as may emerge through the General Household Survey, provide another perspective on morbidity rates. This survey collects data on such topics as the occurrence of chronic and acute illnesses, consultations with doctors, smoking habits, medications and the like. From a medical perspective these data are often described as limited, since they rely on self-diagnosis and an individual's memories of events. That different actors should construct sickness in different ways is not, however, a limitation. A lay person's interpretations may not fit neatly into biomedical disease categorisations, but they are just as, if not more, valid in the determination of the morbidity with which any population is burdened. In addition, there is no evidence available that actually supports the biomedical view that lay people are less able than qualified professionals to diagnose and accurately record their sickness episodes. In fact, there is some research that indicates that health professionals are much less able in this respect (Strong and Davis, 1976). Another national source of information which may provide a more comprehensive perspective on sickness throughout the community was contained for the first time in the 1991 census, which included a question about long-term illness.

More recently, several initiatives have been launched to collect both morbidity and mortality data in association with the *Health of the Nation* strategy and targets (Department of Health, 1992a). The *Public Health Common Data Set* (Department of Health, 1992c,d, 1993e) includes both baseline data for 1992 and subsequent monitoring data which were first released in 1993. A comparative data set provides Health Authorities with past mortality trends, geographic variations and local trends. In addition, new health surveys for 1991 and 1992 (Department of Health, 1993f, 1994b) have been undertaken on aspects of health relevant to one key area – cardiovascular disease. These reported the prevalence of cardiovascular disease and examined the risk factors associated with it. Specific data were obtained on obesity and blood pressure. It is intended that in future years the content of these surveys may change to cover other key areas. The prevalence of mental illness and the factors associated with its emergence are also being determined by the OPCS *National Psychiatric Morbidity Survey*.

In summary, it is clear that both the sources of information about disease and health within a population and the systems for collecting such information are diverse. At the present time none seems either comprehensive or representative of the diverse sets of views through which health and sickness may be constructed by either society or its individual members. Particular data – population, mortality or morbidity – provide a particular picture. Each type of data has its advantages and disadvantages both in terms of compilation and usage. This latter topic will be more fully explored in Chapter 5, while some further consideration of how disease and health are measured within populations will continue below.

MEASURING HEALTH AND DISEASE IN POPULATIONS

Measuring the frequency of disease/illness

In everyday conversations nurses and doctors often discuss the probability of certain events in words. For example, 'most' women spend longer in labour in their first pregnancy than in subsequent confinements; urinary tract infections 'often' occur in patients who are catheterised; patients 'sometimes' reject their 'named nurse'. Substituting words for numbers in this way is convenient, but not very precise. This is because different people ascribe different meanings to commonly used words. Fletcher *et al.* (1988) cite the example of patients who assigned widely different probabilities (from 0.35 to 1.0) to the term 'usually'. It is clear therefore that estimates of probability are more accurately described by numbers. Estimates of how common certain events are govern much clinical practice. Decisions are made according to the likelihood of certain outcomes. If we use a clean but unsterile dressing on an intravenous access site, how likely is it that infection might occur? If infection occurs, how likely is it that the patient will suffer complications? And so on.

Relevant measures of frequency are usually expressed as fractions or proportions, which are commonly termed **rates**. Rates are the basic unit of measurement when studying disease in populations. Rates consist of three elements:

- the **numerator**, which is the number of people in a population who experience the event of interest
- the **denominator**, which is the total number of people in the population, i.e. the population at risk of the event
- the **time period** over which the events of interest took place

Epidemiology is concerned with making comparisons between populations. The use of a rate allows valid comparisons to be made between these populations. For most purposes it is insufficient to have information only about the absolute number of events occurring in two or more populations, although sometimes this may be helpful for planning purposes. A survey of the provision of urethral catheters (Mulhall *et al.*, 1992) illustrates this point. The study noted that several wards which ordered catheters directly from central stores held excessively large numbers. These figures were, however, only meaningful in relation to the rate at which patients in these wards were catheterised. Thus in the urological ward, where the rate of catheterisations was high, a large stock of catheters would be acceptable, whereas in the day ward, where the rate was low, storing excess catheters would be an unnecessary expense and could lead to stock going out of date before it could be used. In other words, it is necessary to have information about relative size when comparing two populations.

Three types of rate are commonly quoted in the demographic and epidemiological literature, particularly in connection with mortality. These are **crude rates**, **specific rates** and **standardised rates**. The crude rate, as it implies, refers to the entire population of the area under consideration, say the mortality rate for North Thames Regional Health Authority. This rate is readily calculated, but provides little information on other important characteristics of the population; for example, the age and social class structure remain unknown.

Specific rates address this by measuring the number of events occurring in a subgroup of the population – for example the mortality rate of males in social class I in two different districts.

A useful summary measure, however, is contained in the standardised rate, which takes account of the structure of two populations. Thus a standard age-specific death rate can be applied to the study population to determine how many deaths would have been expected to occur if the study population experience was the same as the standard experience. The number of actual or observed deaths in the study population is then determined, and the ratio of these two (observed deaths/expected deaths)× 100% provides the **standardised mortality ratio**. This figure provides an easily understood value since ratios over 100% in the study population indicate an unfavourable mortality experience, and those below 100% a favourable outcome.

Many illnesses do not result in death and cannot therefore be described using mortality data. Two rates that are commonly used to describe morbidity are **prevalence** and **incidence** (see also Chapter 1). It is important to distinguish between these terms, which, outside epidemiology, have frequently been applied incorrectly. Mixing or comparing data for incidence with those that indicate prevalence will result in errors of logic (Last, 1987).

Prevalence is the proportion of a defined population who possess a particular condition at a given point in time (point prevalence). Period prevalence refers to the fraction of a population who possess the condition over a specified period of time. Prevalence thus measures all cases existing either at one point in time or over a period of time. It is thus a static measure and strictly speaking should not be referred to as a rate. An easy way of understanding prevalence is to consider it as a 'snapshot' of the given population. If at the beginning of 1995 a practice nurse had 100 patients who attended a well woman clinic and four of them were found to be suffering from vaginal candidosis, then the prevalence of patients with candidosis attending that clinic would be 4% at that point in time. Thus prevalence is affected not just by how many new cases arise, but also by the duration of a condition. Of the four patients above some might have had candidosis for several weeks or months and some might just have developed it.

In contrast, incidence is the proportion of a population who are initially free of the condition who develop it over a specified period of time. Thus the numerator in incidence is the number of new cases occurring in the time period, and the denominator is all susceptible people present at the start of that time period. Continuing with the example of the practice nurse above, and assuming that the patients attending the clinic remain the same, suppose that over the coming year (1995) in two of the four patients the candidosis resolved, and in the remaining two the infection remained. In addition, three other patients developed candidosis. What would be the point prevalence of candidosis on 31 December 1995 and the incidence in 1995? The numerator for the point prevalence would be 5 (since two of the original sufferers were infection-free and three new cases arose) and the denominator remains as 100. Thus the point prevalence would be 5/100. To calculate the incidence of vaginal candidosis, only the 96 women free from infection at the start of the period are considered. Three new cases developed, and thus the incidence is 3/96. Note that this model does not take account of cases which might resolve and then reappear within the year. Figure 4.1 illustrates this example.

Prevalence rates may be calculated by a single survey of a group containing cases and non-cases – a prevalence survey (see Chapter 1). They are mainly useful in planning the allocation of health service resources, since they indicate the amount of illness requiring care. Conditions with a low incidence, e.g. chronic renal failure, may become important problems if their duration is long and their call on resources is high. As described in Chapter 1, incidence can only be measured by a cohort study which monitors the emergence of the condition of interest in a susceptible population over time. The time element is essential to the calculation of incidence. Thus incidence rates provide an estimate of the risk of a condition developing and are useful in aetiological studies which search for the determinants or causes of ill health.

The discussion above underlines why it is important to understand the difference between incidence and prevalence, since these two rates provide the answer to two different questions: 'At what rate do new cases of the condition arise in a population over time?' (incidence) and 'What proportion of people in the population have the condition?' (prevalence).

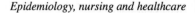

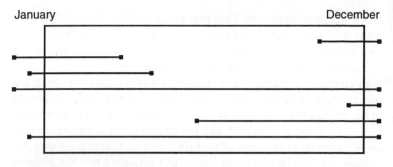

Duration of infection
Point prevalence January 1995 = 4/100
Point prevalence December 1995 = 5/100
Incidence in 1995 = 3/96

Figure 4.1 *Occurrence of vaginal candidosis in 100 clients attending a well woman clinic.*

Two other rates are sometimes used in epidemiology: the **case fatality rate** and the **attack rate**. The case fatality rate is a form of cumulative incidence which measures the proportion of people with a condition who die from it in a defined period after diagnosis. This rate is only meaningful if cases are followed from diagnosis to death or recovery. In fact, the case fatality rate is not a rate at all, since it does not measure the rate per unit of time at risk at which death occurs. The attack rate is most often used in epidemics, and again it is a cumulative incidence which indicates the rate of occurrence in a given population observed for a limited amount of time.

Making sense of prevalence and incidence

The denominator

The above underlines the importance of distinguishing between incidence data and prevalence data, but the way in which the cases and populations within these rates are defined is also crucial to any clear understanding of what these figures represent. One of the most important tasks in epidemiology is the choice of an appropriate denominator. In fact, sometimes the denominator is never included in statements about health risks – the case of the 'floating numerator' (Victora, 1993). Floating numerators are characterised by such statements as 'Most accidents in young children occur at home'. Obviously, young children spend most of their time in the home, but this in itself does not make it a riskier place than, for example, the local park. What is missing is a denominator that would give these statements a measure of relative risk. Three denominators are commonly used in epidemiology to measure disease frequency:

(a) the total number of people in a study
(b) the number of people in the study who do not have the condition of interest at a certain point in time
(c) the number of people at risk of the condition multiplied by the time for which each remains at risk

For most purposes, (a) will be used as the denominator in prevalence rates and (b) the denominator in incidence rates (see the example above of the well woman clinic). However, when people are followed over time (as in a cohort study) to determine incidence it is clear that the numbers at risk will vary. Some people will die from causes other than the condition of interest, and some will move and be lost to follow-up. To allow for these discrepancies, another measure, termed the **incidence rate**, has been developed. Its denominator is (c) – person time units. The incidence rate is the number of cases in a defined period divided by the sum of the time periods at risk for all the individuals in the population. Time units are expressed as perhaps 1 person-year or 1 person-month. So 6 person years might represent 6 people followed for one year, or 3 people followed for 2 years. Incidence rates are particularly useful in aetiological studies of chronic diseases, where the incubation period of the disease may be longer than the period of observation in the study.

Two other important points about denominators require mentioning. Firstly, the denominator should only be composed of those who are susceptible to the condition counted in the numerator. Thus a valid denominator for studies of the prevalence of uterine cancer would not only just include women, but only those women who had not had a hysterectomy. This point is discussed by Clark and Cullum (1992) in their study of pressure sore prevalence and the supply of pressure-redistributing mattresses. They state that the denominator used in calculating the prevalence of pressure sores should be the population *at risk* as defined by the Norton Score (Norton *et al.*, 1962), not the total population studied. Thus although they surveyed all patients in the seven hospitals of one District Health Authority, i.e. 866 subjects, they contend that only those at risk, i.e. 294, should be used to estimate prevalence. When this method of calculation was used the prevalence in their study changed from 10.3% to 21.4%. This highlights aspects of the second point, namely that the denominator should reflect the population of interest. Usually for epidemiologists this is the total population in one geographical area, but for practitioners the relevant populations are more likely to be groups with specific clinical conditions presenting at a limited number of clinical facilities.

The question here centres on the generalisability of rates. Thus cases seen at, for example, a tertiary referral centre are unlikely to be the same either in terms of disease severity, treatment or outcome as cases of the same condition who are cared for by GPs. When using prevalence and incidence rates in clinical practice it is thus essential firstly to ensure that the denominators chosen are meaningful in terms of the population described, and secondly that this population is similar to one's own patients or clients.

The numerator

It would seem simple enough to define the 'cases' that should be included in the numerator, but several problems may arise. The classification of ill persons into groups and the definition of the boundaries between those groups is termed **nosology**. The International Classification of Diseases provides one such nosology, upon which much epidemiological work is based. For example, the causes of death in the returns sent to OPCS are coded according to this system. However, as Last (1987, p. 39) notes, 'The classification of disease entities,... has hardy changed since 1855 when William Farr and Marc D'Espigne presented their ideas to the Second International Statistical Congress in Paris'. Serious deficiencies and inaccuracies have become apparent over this time, but perhaps of more importance is the recognition that a conceptual change in its framework is required. It is planned that the tenth revision, for use beyond this millennium, must adopt an integrated classification more consonant with present-day conceptions of health and illness and detailing not only symptoms but reasons for encounters with providers of healthcare, complaints and problems (White, 1984).

Epidemiologists are most often concerned with determining which people in a population have a certain condition, at whatever stage it might be (subclinical, fatal, in remission, as a carrier state and so on). This gradient of disease may be identified in some conditions by laboratory investigations, but for certain chronic diseases, such as multiple sclerosis, no comparable procedures exist. In contrast with the epidemiologist, the clinician is most often dealing with conditions which have produced discernible signs and symptoms that will have some effect, such as death or disability. Explicit diagnostic criteria may be used to define cases, but often they are so detailed and specific as to exclude most people who would, in ordinary clinical practice, be considered to have the condition.

It can be seen, therefore, that any valid interpretation of rates is strongly dependent upon knowing the basis on which the cases included have been defined. Studies need to adhere to a definition of the case that is predefined. In practice this is not always easy. Glenister (1991) describes the lengthy and difficult discussions (eight draft papers) to reach a consensus agreement on definitions before her study of different methods of surveillance of hospital-acquired infections could proceed. Additionally, if certain laboratory tests are required to 'prove the case' then bias may be introduced if the test is performed only in specialised centres, thus excluding certain parts of the population who would not be cared for in these locations. Similarly, persons succumbing to rapidly fatal conditions, such as myocardial infarction, might die before the test necessary for inclusion as a 'case' was performed. These practical difficulties affecting the numerator would seriously bias any measurement of the distribution of such conditions.

A 'case' may also be defined in different ways according to perspective. It has been noted how clinical cases may differ from epidemiological cases, but lay perspectives will add another dimension. Sanders (1962) reports the differences between lay and professional definitions of various conditions in a population interviewed at home. Wide variations in definition occurred: for example, just over 2% of people reported that they had heart disease, but examination by a physician revealed that four times this number would have clinically defined heart disease.

This returns us to the central debate first raised in Chapter 2 as to the classification of disease and sickness. The question is, who should define a case? Lay definitions are just as, or perhaps more, valid than biomedical definitions. Certainly the use to which the information from any study will be put may determine how and by whom a case is best defined. This is particularly pertinent where epidemiological studies are used in the planning of healthcare. It raises thorny issues as to how decisions concerning, for example, the allocation of resources should be made. The *Health of the Nation* initiatives have at least recognised that consumer perspectives on, for example, outcome evaluation are important. However, strategic planning and allocation of health service resources have seldom taken account of lay perspectives. Where epidemiology purports to be concerned with the assessment of needs and how they should be met, much greater emphasis is required in determining whose need and the optimal strategies for meeting them. Determining the numerator in prevalence and incidence studies forms part of these arguments and further discussion of this topic occurs in Chapter 5.

THE SOCIAL AND POLITICAL DIMENSIONS OF HEALTH INFORMATION

The final section of this chapter is concerned with an exploration of how health statistics may be affected by factors which go beyond the presentation of seemingly objective numbers and percentages. For Western societies, founded as they are on a strong notion of scientific rationalism, statistics can prove overwhelmingly compelling. Add to this the aversion that many nurses and doctors have to utilising or understanding numerical data and it may be seen that enormous scope exists for intended or spurious statistical 'deceptions'. Without the skills or insights to challenge such statistics, nurses will be impotent in the face of arguments built on this type of data. This is not to say that health information statistics are wrong or dangerous, but to emphasise that certain factors beyond the data set itself must be considered when examining its validity for guiding healthcare practices or policies. This section will consider three aspects of health data: the hidden aspects of data set construction; the social construction of data; and finally the suppression of data.

The hidden aspects of data sets

Information about the health of communities may be collected and analysed on a routine basis or may be derived from specially conducted surveys. There is no doubt that this information is vital to the effective planning of health services. However, the use of such data by either practitioners or managers should be governed by the recognition of two features which may limit or misconstrue interpretation. Firstly, statistical data, particularly to those unfamiliar with its construction, can be distorted and manipulated to present a particular 'picture'. Secondly, the collection and construction of data sets are open to sociocultural influences from the first question which prompts their initiation through to their use in the healthcare arena. The old maxim that 'there are three kinds of lies: lies, damned lies, and statistics' (Disraeli) therefore perhaps merits more serious recognition than it usually receives.

It is not possible here to discuss in any depth the different ways in which statistical data may be misrepresented. The discussion above concerning 'floating numerators' provides a simple example of where the lack of a relevant comparison measure, i.e. the denominator, can render a statistic meaningless. Other commonly quoted examples include graphs where the proportions of the axes have been changed (either extended to overemphasise or compacted to underemphasise the results), or where the bottom of the graph is removed again to emphasise a particular point. These are ploys, and as such relatively easy to uncover; other manipulations, which may involve sophisticated 'number crunching' using statistical computer packages are less easily discerned. On other occasions the statistical rigour behind sets of figures is questionable. Was the sample size large enough to draw the stated conclusions (see Chapter 1 for Type I and II errors)? Did the basis of recording information (perhaps the definition of cases) change?

Perhaps the most sensible advice when attempting to recognise sound and usable data is to shed the terror of numbers (which seems inherent in most of us) and to scrutinise the information carefully for obvious manipulations and for statements which at face value to do fit with our common understandings. For example, at the beginning of the chapter it was mentioned that the forecasting of population trends was a relatively hit and miss affair. In some senses life experience predicts that this is likely to be the case. The extrapolation to future rates of mortality, migration and fertility seems a difficult if not impossible task. The value accorded to these statistics should therefore be restricted – to a practitioner, indeed to anyone, they have little face value.

Health data, indeed any data, are not produced in a vacuum devoid from the factors that are shaping other aspects of political and economic life. As Dale *et al.* (1988, p. 25) tellingly note, 'the construction of a data-base is a socially negotiated exercise'. Recognising rigorous data that are relevant to one's own practice therefore requires some examination of the foundation through which the data set has been produced. It is helpful in this context to realise that data are produced rather than collected. Interpretations will therefore vary according to perspective. Any claim that data collected from interviews, observations or surveys is objective cannot therefore be upheld (Dale *et al.*, 1988). Some simple questions should guide an interrogation of the data's heritage and origins: Who defined the topic described by the statistics?; Does the information set out to provide evidence to substantiate a particular viewpoint?; Whose definitions are used? (Adams *et al.*, 1994).

Take the example of governmental statistics, which are after all collected by the government. Questions in government-sponsored surveys, such as the General Household Survey or the new Health Surveys, will be modified or omitted according to the current expediencies of policymakers. The prevailing politico-economic environment will shape the data and cannot be ignored by the user of such statistics.

How the data were collected is also important. Some of the problems related to the collection of mortality data were mentioned at the start of the chapter. In addition, the method of collection – questionnaire, interview, independent observation – will influence the type of material that is produced. Government-sponsored surveys produce highly standardised material, but the structured interviews used to generate the data will be unable to capture more complex issues concerning, say, health beliefs or the inner meanings that people attach to them.

As a final point it is also worth noting that data that are collected routinely are particularly dependent upon those who are required to record it. In general, healthcare practitioners do not lay great store by collecting and recording routine data. An unrelated but apposite anecdote illustrates this point. 'A judge in India once told a young British civil servant, "When you are a bit older you will not quote Indian statistics with that assurance. The government are very keen on amassing statistics – they collect them, add them, raise them to the *n*th power, take the cube root and produce wonderful diagrams. But what you must never forget is that every one of those figures comes in the first instance from the *chowty dar* (village watchman), who just puts down what he damn pleases"' (Huff, 1973). While not wishing to accuse either the government or the professions of such calumny, it is evident that a flavour of the above story does not sit amiss with much of the current activity in the health services.

The social construction of data

The previous section noted how social and politico-economic factors may affect how, when, why and in what manner statistics about health may be produced. From another perspective, however, the sociocultural environment may construct categories or problems at certain times and in certain places. In other words, health 'problems' and the statistics which surround them are just as much a product of society as they are of physiological or pathological processes. Two examples will be discussed – stress and perinatal mortality.

The concept of stress is familiar to professionals and lay people alike: it is understood by all and yet defined satisfactorily by none. A plethora of disciplines – psychology, psychiatry, medicine, sociology, ergonomics, anthropology and pharmacology – have studied stress, each its their own objectives and particular methodologies. Between 1987 and 1992 the psychological literature alone, cites 10,385 articles related to this subject. As Cox (1992, p. 25) notes, 'the varied influx of workers into stress research has resulted in a grand alliance and confusion of terminology'.

The current discourse on stress pervades both the medical and popular literature. However, Pollock (1988, p. 381) argues that stress is 'not something that is naturally occurring in the world, but a manufactured concept which has now become a social fact'. It appears that the discovery and elaboration of stress as a theoretical concept has parallelled its diffusion and acceptance in society.

Stress is constantly 'called on' in contemporary society, but it is also attached to a morally constructed environment. The popular discourse on stress shares many of the assumptions with the biomedical discourse. Stress in both arenas is taken as a *real* concept, which does, however, vary widely. Young (1980) expounds on the ideology of the stress discourse. He suggests that the congruence of middle-class American beliefs about social nature and the ideology of stress legitimises and verifies the concept in many minds. Pollock (1988, p. 387) adds that stress can be used to 'locate the source of responsibility for illness in the individual, or a pathogenic social structure'. Stress may thus support ideological views concerning the social order, an individual's 'place', and the locus of responsibility for healthcare.

It is apparent then that although the precise nature and aetiology of stress eludes definition, and the relationship between stress and illness is far from clear, this concept has grasped both the popular and scientific imaginations. Modern industrial society has adopted the notion of stress and transformed it into an illness. The medical and lay conceptions of stress overlap and are mutually reinforcing. Foucault (1973) states that 'There is... a spontaneous and deeply rooted convergence between the requirements of political ideology and those of medical technology', and in its ideological component the stress discourse may indicate this convergence (Pollock, 1988). The example of stress illustrates therefore how certain health conditions may be constructed in specific ways by society to meet particular individual, cultural or politico-ideological agendas. In this way it can be seen that health information statistics are not necessarily neutral and objective measures, but reflect the current sociocultural milieu.

In a similar but slightly different vein David Armstrong (1986) discusses how infant mortality has 'emerged' as a socio-medical problem during the 20th century. The Registration Act of 1834 required that the cause of death be entered into public records. This introduced the idea of a pathological (rather than a natural) cause of death in the form of disease, and represented an extension of the new pathological medicine into the public domain. Death no longer came from the world of nature external to the body, but from the domain of pathology within. It was not until 1877, however, that infant deaths were reported as the infant mortality rate (IMR). The creation of the IMR, Armstrong contends, suggests two things – a social awareness of infant deaths and the recognition of the infant as a discrete entity.

By the early 20th century infant deaths had been transposed from a biological problem to a social problem which warranted surveillance and intervention through various welfare schemes. The problem of infant mortality was thereby invented through the statistics used to describe it. Furthermore, its conceptualisation as a social problem validated its use (which continues to this day) as an indicator of the well-being and health of communities.

By the mid-1950s the first year of life of a child's life had been segmented into temporal spaces (the perinatal period, the neonatal period etc.) which delineated the infant's **physical** identity. However, by this time the infant had also acquired a **social** identity. Furthermore, Armstrong argues that the conceptual space of this social identity was not bounded by the application of objective epidemiological techniques as might first appear, since such neutrality assumes that the infant had an identity separate from the techniques used to explore it. But the construction of infancy was in fact an arbitrary convention driven by the methodological techniques that created it. In other words, the attributes of infancy can be seen as a reflection of the techniques that first brought the child into the medical perception. For medicine the infant has an *a priori* existence, and yet it is the statistical techniques that created this object and brought into the medical gaze. The infant had no existence before the statistical analysis of deaths in the first year of life was imposed. Furthermore, once neonatal mortality had been identified as a problem of social and domestic influences (such as nutrition, domestic hygiene and educational background), its biological underpinning could be imposed to create a moral and social order surrounding the standard of family life and motherhood. This discussion culminates in the question of what exactly the official statistics regarding infant mortality represent. From a medical perspective the figures represent 'reality' as portrayed through the assignment of individual deaths to specific categories. This is despite the fact that the rules governing assignment have changed over the years. The statistics do not, however, so much represent reality as the classification system on which they are founded.

The two examples provided in this section illustrate the importance of bringing a critical eye to bear on health statistics and information. Not only must such data be scrutinised for its statistical soundness and meaningful application, but the underpinnings in its creation must be unravelled. Classifications and categories may become so firmly entrenched that their underlying frameworks are rarely questioned. Greater attention needs to be paid to the wider context in which such health statistics are created and the particular images that they sustain.

The suppression of data

The suppression of health-related data is an historic and ongoing phenomenon that manifests itself in two forms: firstly, the conscious containment of data that would be damaging to certain groups or bodies such as the government, and secondly the subconscious repression that may emerge from the different perspectives through which different groups view problems and their solution. Although neither case is desirable, the conscious repression of data is somewhat easier to discern, even if it remains as intractable to reform as subconscious repression.

The restriction of the report from the Black working party (Black, 1980) into the differential health experiences associated with different social classes must stand as one of the most infamous examples of the conscious suppression of health-related data. The information that there were dramatic and increasing social class inequalities was highly unpalatable to the Conservative government's contention that a resurgence of British capitalism would result in universal and equal benefits. Contrary to normal practice this report was not published through HMSO.

Further restrictions were to occur. Data appearing after the 1981 census in the *Decennial Supplement on Occupational Mortality* would have provided further evidence as to whether the trends noted in the Black Report were persisting. However, when the *Supplement* appeared the analysis by social class had been removed, to be available by microfiche only at a cost of £40 plus VAT (the actual report costing only £9.50). Subsequently, the author of the report resigned his post and published an article which reported that the difference in death rates in manual and non-manual workers had increased in the previous ten years (Marmot and McDowell, 1986).

Other classic examples of the suppression of health statistics are to be found in the opposition to the work of the National Advisory Committee on Nutritional Education (NACNE) by the British Nutritional Foundation, which is largely sponsored by the food industry (Thunhurst, 1991). The general concerns about official statistics are perhaps epitomised by the convening of a meeting of the Royal Statistical Society in December 1989 to review and discuss the 'Integrity and Validity of Official Statistics'. The outcome of this was the setting up of a working party to 'provide an independent review of the criteria and mechanisms for monitoring the integrity and adequacy of, and public confidence in, official statistics'.

The unconscious suppression of data about health is, as mentioned above, more difficult to uncover. Relevant here is the discussion in the previous section concerning the construction of data sets. Who asks the questions? Which definitions do they use? How does the analysis proceed? Have subtle and covert construction of health problems such as stress and infant mortality occurred?. Epidemiological information does not always speak for itself (in fact it rarely does). Different groups will approach data with different priorities and perspectives. Policy formulators may differ in their interpretations of health statistics and thus in the interventions that they may recommend as a result. These differences are not so much overt but subsumed within a certain 'mind-set'. Once problems are defined in particular ways it may become peculiarly difficult to perceive them in different ways. The construction of conceptual models restricts the information that may emerge to that which is consonant with the prevailing set of assumptions on which the model is based. Information 'which is not congruent with the prevailing outlook tends to be ignored, re-interpreted, suppressed or even at times condemned' (Levine and Lilienfeld, 1987, p. 13).

This chapter has covered a wide range of territory and utilised a number of differing frameworks in an attempt to provide an informative and yet critical review of health information and statistics. The pragmatic aspects of health data and their collection have been provided, since this is a basic set of knowledge with which nursing must become familiar to fight its own corner in the new NHS. More and more government directives and initiatives are framed on such 'hard' data. To be familiar with and to understand the concepts and terminology, and the pitfalls to their use, is essential. The final section has given some indications of other aspects of health information which go beyond the face value of facts and figures. An appreciation of these political and social dimensions is equally as important as, for example, understanding how prevalence is calculated. Indeed, it is probably more important, for it brings into the consciousness an attitude that is frequently lacking when faced with sets of graphs and figures. In Western societies hard numerical data has a particular grasp on our belief systems, often extending way beyond the statistics themselves. Nursing needs to be aware of this aspect of health services culture in order that such data may be productively used or adapted/discarded where its construction is found to be wanting.

CHAPTER FIVE

Planning healthcare services and epidemiology

The recent restructuring of the health service and the emergence of the internal market have precipitated major changes in the philosophical and organisational character of the National Health Service (NHS). Quality assurance and evaluation programmes are being developed to maximise the delivery of care to patients, who have been transformed into clients. Planning healthcare within this new environment demands a greater emphasis on the development of good information systems and on appropriate health need and health gain measures. Indeed, such initiatives are integral to the health targets outlined in *The Health of the Nation* (Department of Health, 1992a). But how are these initiatives to be realised? For many the answer lies in epidemiology. Several of the methods traditionally used in epidemiological studies could provide the evidence to guide the strategic planning of health services, including the role of nursing within these.

The significant effect which the changes in the organisational structure of the NHS since the early 1970s have had on nurses' work (see Chapter 3) cannot have left any in the profession in doubt of the need to respond rapidly to new initiatives with knowledge and confidence. To fail in this respect is to allow other more powerful groups to dictate, rather than debate, how nurses and nursing should be managed and organised. If, as is undoubtedly the case, epidemiology is going to be used as the linchpin in many of the ensuing debates concerning the resourcing of the NHS and the distribution of those resources, then nursing must become familiar with epidemiology – its principles, practices, pitfalls and dilemmas. From a firm basis of knowledge, nursing will be able to back up or refute the arguments put forward by others, and in addition, formulate its own strategies within a similar framework.

Planning and evaluation form a considerable part of health service administration. Several books (for example Ham (1982), Butler and Vaile (1985) and Abel-Smith (1994)) and an extensive literature produced by the government (for example the Black Report (Black, 1980) and the Körner Report on health statistics (Department of Health and Social Security, 1982)) are the focus of this subject. Several aspects of planning have been addressed already in previous chapters. The reorganisation of the health service (Chapter 3), the use of health information (Chapter 4) and the section on surveillance and control in Chapter 6 are some examples. This chapter will continue the theme of examining particular aspects of planning where epidemiology may make a contribution.

Planning is a continuous process which, for the NHS, should involve managers, planners and the direct deliverers of the service – the healthcare professionals. The task is to formulate programmes within the framework of both national policies and local needs using available resources. Planning aims to ensure the provision of necessary services of acceptable quality at the right place, and at the right time (Abel-Smith, 1994). Successful planning is dependent on two main exigencies:

- the availability of accurate and adequate information
- an organisational structure which both values planning and ensures that strategies are implemented and evaluated

Donaldson and Donaldson (1993) note that the quality of the former has been singularly lacking within the NHS, but suggest that new efforts being introduced to improve the quality of routinely collected data will alleviate this problem. In addition, they propose that the 1984 reorganisation has led the way to ensuring that strategic planning is given greater priority. The normative approach to planning that prevailed until recently in the NHS produced guidelines from 'outside and above' as to the nature and extent that services at local level should take. Increasingly, service planning is being organised through the estimation of the need for services among particular populations and the extent to which this need is being met. The central objective of this planning is 'to identify and meet the needs of a population in the most efficient and effective way' (Donaldson and Donaldson, 1993, p. 187). Recent political initiatives – in particular the white papers on hospital services and community care (Department of Health, 1989b,c) – laid the foundation for this trend. The recommendations of these papers are enshrined in the NHS and Community Care Act (1991), which places a statutory requirement on District Health Authorities to assess the healthcare needs of their populations.

This then is the pragmatic face of health service planning, but contained within it are certain principles that perhaps deserve rather more thought than they have so far received. The changes brought about over the last ten years in the NHS have not occurred in isolation. They are located within a wider ideological, economic and socio-political framework, which although apposite to the discussion of other subjects tackled in this book is particularly pertinent to the planning and provision of services, for service provision and structuring lies at the heart of the NHS and thus exerts a considerable influence upon the activities that are subsumed within its auspices. Debates about planning and provision cannot be limited to simplistic statistical arguments over the definition of healthcare problems and the identification of strategies that effectively and efficiently meet these needs. The issues go beyond this to such questions as: What do we expect a modern health service to provide? How do we allocate limited resources? What needs to be done in the wider context to improve the nation's health? These are questions which are edged to the margin and rarely addressed (Ranade, 1994). Alongside this are other deeper philosophical questions surrounding the 'principles' of the NHS – principles that are frequently articulated, but rarely defined with any precision.

These are important issues for, as mentioned in the preface, epidemiology is gaining increased prominence within a culture that requires objective measures of the health profile of populations. Calls are being made at both a governmental and local level for more accurate epidemiological information to measure patient need and outcomes (Department of Health, 1994c). Indeed, a new Central Health Monitoring Unit has been set up by the Department of Health to provide epidemiological data to underpin the formulation and implementation of policy. While the role of epidemiology in effective healthcare planning is not disputed, before we rush headlong down this particular path it is important to take a hard look at the foundations upon which some of the principles guiding this work are based.

This chapter is divided into two sections. The first describes the 'conventional' account of how and where epidemiology may make the maximum contribution in the planning of an effective health service. As stated at the beginning of the chapter, healthcare planning covers a wide remit, and a single chapter can only provide an indication to the area. Traditionally epidemiology has played a major role in public health. This chapter on planning therefore focuses on the changing emphasis within public health following the Acheson Report (Department of Health and Social Security 1988). This ushered in the era of the 'new public health' (see Chapter 1) which stresses the importance of the structural and environmental causes of ill health, and emphasises the participation of communities in determining health needs and the strategies to meet them. Some of the topics to be covered include such issues as defining populations; determining their patterns of 'disease'; and the provision and evaluation of apposite and adequate services. The second section of the chapter will fundamentally challenge the first by posing the question: is rational planning possible? It will explore such areas as health need, health gain and quality under an overlying theme of questioning what the purpose of the NHS is.

HEALTH PLANNING – THE CONVENTIONAL APPROACH

Simplistically, planning for the provision of health services may be viewed as a three-stage process which determines:

1. What the healthcare 'problems' of a population are.
2. How services should be arranged to address these problems.
3. How services should be evaluated.

Epidemiology has a considerable part to play in all of these processes. In Chapter 1, epidemiology was defined as 'the study of the distribution and determinants of health related states and events in defined populations, and the application of this study to the control of health problems' (Last, 1987, p. 29). Thus epidemiological methods may be used to quantify the nature and extent of healthcare 'problems' in defined populations (process 1), and to determine those strategies that might be most effective and efficient in controlling these 'problems' (process 2). Epidemiological methods are also useful for evaluating the differential outcome of strategies (process 3), such as different ways of delivering care, which may be instituted as a result of planning activities. The evaluation of healthcare technologies has assumed a priority in recent governmental policy initiatives (Department of Health, 1992b) spawned by *The Health of the Nation* (Department of Health, 1992a). Chapter 6 provides a wide discussion of health technology assessment (HTA) in nursing, and the role of epidemiological methods within this.

Determining healthcare problems

Defining the population and the environment

The first step in determining the healthcare problems in any community is the description of the characteristics of the population involved. For a hospital-based nurse this population would encompass the patients and staff and also the wider population from which these are drawn. In terms of public health, however, the community would normally include the whole population in, for example, a District Health Authority.

The study of populations of people is termed demography. Demographers determine the absolute numbers of people living in a particular geographical area, and other related parameters, such as the age structure, fertility rate, mortality rate and birth rate, of the population. The data that demographers use are mostly derived from censuses and the registration of births and deaths. Chapter 4 provides a full description of these statistics, including some of the problems and biases inherent in their collection and use. Thus although demography is not essentially a health science, it provides the data that are necessary for this first stage of planning health services by establishing a foundation for further development. Adequate and appropriate services can only be estimated on the basis of firm data concerning the characteristics of the population in question. Estimates of overall numbers of people are necessary for planning services that all the population requires (for example, access to dental or GP services), while specific sections of the population, such as pre-school children, need to be identified to determine the need for particular services, which in this case might be immunisation programmes.

Any thorough assessment of potential health problems must also include a description of the environment of the community. In public health terms this needs to cover such items as the physical and geographical characteristics of the neighbourhood; transportation; the pattern of industry and commerce; leisure facilities; religious affiliations; healthcare facilities; and voluntary organisations. These characteristics of the environment may directly affect health status. For example, a raised level of unemployment may result in high rates of depression, suicide, violent crime and chemical substance abuse. Alternatively, the environment may indirectly affect health through the restriction on the ability of individuals to access and gain maximum benefit from health services. For example, poor public transport facilities may result in a failure to attend for follow-up visits at hospitals. A knowledge of the environment of communities is essential as an indication of both the type of problem that may be prevalent and its potential aetiology.

Patterns of mortality and morbidity: what are the important problems?

The pattern of mortality and morbidity in the population as ascertained through epidemiological techniques will provide the next layer of data necessary to determine which issues are particular problems for this community. These data will normally be presented as frequency counts and prevalence and incidence rates. Although mortality rates should be relatively accurate, problems in the coding of such data, particularly for the cause of death, are inevitable given the present system of reporting. Chapter 4 discusses this in some detail and also notes the relative paucity of information available concerning morbidity. Rates need to be calculated for several years to study trends over time and to examine whether genuine changes are occurring. Other epidemiological characteristics which might be included are survival rates by condition, the rate of concomitant psychological and physiological impairments, and the level of compliance with different treatment regimens. Although the addition of this type of data is desirable, it is frequently unavailable unless a specific study has been conducted.

Once mortality and morbidity rates have been ascertained, a more difficult task evolves which concerns the decision over which conditions should be considered a 'problem'. For health planning purposes a problem has been defined by Bales (1983) after Valenis (1992, p. 401) as 'any deviation from a standard, desired, or expected state of affairs'. Deviations from the normal rate may be determined by comparing present rates either with previous rates for the same community, or with concurrent rates within other communities. When using comparisons between communities, valid inferences are only possible where careful matching of the two populations has occurred. If a comparison with previous rates within the same community is proposed, then any changes in population structure or environmental conditions must be sought before any conclusions may be drawn. Caution is necessary because such changes may give the impression that underlying rates have changed when in fact change may perhaps be due to the new way in which services are provided. For example, the introduction of a new tertiary care facility might attract a greater proportion of severely ill clients to a district, thus elevating the mortality rate for a particular condition.

Although the pattern of disease is less prone to bias in a single country, when comparing it across populations it is important to ascertain whether any differences noted are real. A higher frequency recorded in one area compared with another may not represent a genuine difference in disease rates. Variations in healthcare practice may influence the criteria through which diseases are defined and thus their apparent rates in particular areas (see Chapter 2). Lay definitions and practices regarding consultations will also determine when and from whom people seek help for their condition. Only conditions that come to the attention of the healthcare services are likely to enter the official statistics. This ensures that variations in identifying all cases of the disease will also occur. Official record-gathering systems may also vary in their efficiency across areas, causing a similar effect.

A particular approach to the identification of healthcare 'problems' has been adopted in the UK since 1991. This was initiated by *The Health of the Nation* (Department of Health, 1992a) and is continued within many subsequent documents, such as *One Year On* (Department of Health, 1993g), *Targeting Practice: The Role of Nurses, Midwives and Health Visitors* (Department of Health, 1993c) and *A Vision for the Future: The Nursing, Midwifery and Health Visiting Contribution to Health and Health Care* (Department of Health, 1993b), to name but a few. (No doubt by the time this book is published countless others will have appeared.) The strategy selected five key areas for action with regard to improving health: coronary heart disease and stroke, cancers, mental illness, HIV/AIDS and sexual health, and accidents. Three criteria governed the selection of the key areas (Department of Health, 1992a, p. 8):

- The area should be a major cause of premature death or avoidable ill health.
- Effective interventions should be possible, offering significant scope for improvement in health.
- It should be possible to set objectives and targets, and monitor progress towards them.

Each key area has an associated set of targets (25 in all) concerning improvements in health. For example, in the key area HIV/AIDS and sexual health, one of the targets is 'to reduce the rate of conceptions among the under 16's by at least 50% by the year 2000'. *Public Health Common Data Sets* (Department of Health, 1992c,d, 1993e) have also been established to provide health authorities with a comprehensive and comparative set of data concerning the health of the residents in their areas. Thus mechanisms are rapidly being put in place whereby the extent and distribution of those health problems identified in *The Health of the Nation* strategy may be determined at a national level. More locally, District Health Authorities are determining focus areas under the auspices of *The Health of the Nation* and which identify with the healthcare needs of specific groups (e.g. neonatal and maternal health). Local health needs assessment is proceeding also through the estimation of nursing workload profiles, particularly those of health visitors and district nurses.

Although the white paper noted that other existing areas which were sufficiently well developed, such as food safety and childhood immunisation, should continue to be maintained and built upon, the key areas have come to dominate subsequent policy documents. Thus *Targeting Practice* (Department of Health, 1993c, p. 5) notes that 'The Health of the Nation targets have prompted considerable activity in the refocusing of services' (nursing, midwifery and health visiting). Furthermore the same document defines 'good practice' as embracing the principle that 'objectives and targets are achievable and consistent with 'Health of the Nation' and local targets' (Department of Health, 1993c, p. 8). Similarly, an increasing number of district and regional strategies for health have incorporated *Health of the Nation* targets (Department of Health, 1993g). In some respects, therefore, a hegemonic discourse rooted within a particular governmental policy initiative has emerged to shape the face of much health service planning in the late 1980s and 1990s.

It is appropriate here to mention purchasing. The restructuring of the NHS has opened the opportunity for District Health Authorities and other purchasers of healthcare to shape the pattern of health service provision. Health needs assessment is therefore a key element in purchasing. However, several difficulties, concerning such issues as expert versus lay opinion, intervention versus prevention, and quality of life versus saving life, have been recognised (Heginbotham and Ham, 1992). These fundamental dilemmas of purchasing and needs assessment must be addressed in any attempt to synthesise the priorities of such interested parties as the government, providers, healthcare professionals and the public. The concept of health needs assessment has broadened from a purely disease-oriented approach based on a supply and demand model (National Health Service Management Executive, 1990) to discussions of healthy alliances across healthcare boundaries and between individuals and professionals (National Health Service Management Executive, 1992). However, it is clear that if health needs assessment is to be more than a 'genuflexion to the notion of participation and partnership' (Williams and Popay, 1994b, p. 101), some critical thinking and restructuring of sociocultural boundaries will be required. The issue of individual and community participation in health needs assessment is discussed at greater length later in this chapter.

This section has reviewed some of the more practical aspects involved in determining the health problems of a defined population. It has also noted that many different perspectives may be brought to the consideration of how these 'problems' may be defined. In terms of the public health it is clear that the *Health of the Nation* strategy has evolved as a dominant discourse through which much planning and reorganisation of services – nursing, medical and other – is likely to occur. Thus for the first time in England there is a shared and coherent strategy moulding the shape of future health services. However, this also implies that planning (at least strategic planning) has largely been determined at the centre. Moreover, this central strategy is also upheld by new sets of health statistics (for example, *The Public Health Common Data Set*) that have been developed for just this purpose. At one level this may be viewed as logical and indeed necessary information through which the targets as set may be appraised and monitored. However, at another level these statistical data meet the needs of the policies through which they evolved and thus continue to uphold the dominant discourse about, for example, which healthcare problems are important. This returns us to the central question concerning how and by whom the healthcare problems of a population should be defined. This is a theme which will be further discussed in the last section of this chapter.

Determining strategies to address identified health problems

Healthcare planning may be regarded as an exercise in problem-solving which involves a series of steps towards the solution. Valenis (1992) describes this process in some detail; in summarising her approach, seven main steps may be identified:

- identifying and describing the problem
- listing potential causes
- ranking causes
- determining methods for addressing the causes, and their feasibility
- determining resources
- determining target groups
- choosing a programme

Planning or problem-solving in this way may be conducted by hand using flow charts and decision-making trees or though the use of computer models. For example, Yorkshire Regional Health Authority has developed a computer model that simulates the effect of varying the level of different preventative activities for coronary heart disease. For instance, the model predicts that although improved therapy may reduce the mortality rate, this will be at the cost of increased levels of treatment. However, reducing the attack rate for CHD decreases both treatment levels and death rate.

Much could, and indeed has, been written about the problem-solving approach and its various elements. The comments here confine themselves to illustrating where epidemiology impinges on this process. The previous section discussed the issue of **identifying and describing** health problems and how epidemiology is used to determine and thereby describe the extent of these problems (as incidence, prevalence, attack rates etc.) and their geographical distribution.

Listing and ranking potential causes

Although Chapter 4 highlighted some of the difficulties in identifying and describing information related to health problems (even for data as ostensibly objective and straightforward as mortality rates), listing and ranking the potential causes of health problems is a more difficult endeavour. Much epidemiological research is undertaken to elucidate cause and effect relationships. Possible causes may be gleaned from a review of the literature, which should include a search for factors that may have a role in the development, presence and continuation of the problem. It is important to note, however, that it is not necessary to understand or even know the specific cause of a problem in order to solve it. Chapter 1 noted the case of legionnaire's disease, where the association of this condition with water supplies in large buildings was observed before the aetiological agent (*Legionella pneumophila*) was isolated. Certain control measures, such as the periodic cleaning of air conditioning systems, could therefore be planned prior to knowledge concerning the definitive aetiology of legionnaire's disease being available.

However, the role of any potential factor in causation must be carefully examined, and causation should never be assumed. Any potential factor must be scrutinised using the criteria first outlined by Bradford (see Chapter 1). These criteria, such as temporality and the strength of the association, may be used for evaluating the evidence for causality. This will then form the basis for planning particular activities and programmes to prevent or control the condition. The pitfalls of not following this approach may be illustrated by the case of pap smears for cervical cancer. Many planners have assumed that the problem of reducing deaths from cervical cancer was related to a lack of pap smears. However, without an appropriate epidemiological study it is a false assumption to claim that cervical cancer rates are directly related to the uptake of pap tests. In fact, Martin (1972) reported that 42% of women dying of cervical cancer had had annual pap smears. The major factor leading to the deaths of these women was not therefore a failure to be screened, but errors in the screening procedure itself, such as a failure to follow up suspicious results, lost reports and laboratory errors. A more recent example is the conundrum provided by screening for breast cancer. Although screening rates are improving, mortality from this disease is showing only a small decline.

The major health problems of the 1990s are chronic long-term conditions rather than the acute infectious diseases that taxed the public health pioneers of the 19th century. The identification of planning strategies to reduce or eliminate these health problems is complicated by two factors. Firstly, the aetiology of many chronic conditions is often partially unresolved and is certainly multifactorial. Secondly, the contribution that 'lifestyle' makes in their causation is frequently unclear.

Although for planning purposes it may be helpful to differentiate between classes of causes, such as biological, environmental, educational and administrative, which may all contribute to the existence of a particular health problem, these rarely exist in isolation and are often interdependent. Even within 'classes of cause' interdependence occurs. Take coronary heart disease (CHD): two main biological risk factors for this condition have been proposed – blood pressure and serum cholesterol concentration. These two factors are, however, linked so that the mortality rate from CHD in people with a high cholesterol level almost doubles for those who also have high blood pressure (Nuffield Institute for Health, Centre for Health Economics and Royal College of Physicians, 1993). Other biological risk factors include obesity and diabetes. Furthermore a social/behavioural factor – cigarette smoking – is also a major determinant of CHD.

Ranking these causes in order to plan a public health strategy to reduce deaths from CHD is difficult, although the government white paper confidently states that smoking is responsible for 18% of CHD deaths, and that a reduction of 10% in the average serum cholesterol level might result in a 20–30% reduction in the mortality rate. CHD has been extensively studied over the last twenty years, but for many chronic conditions this type of data is not available. Selecting potential causes for targeting in these cases is more difficult. Moreover, caution needs to be exercised even where seemingly straightforward relationships between biological variables and disease have been established. Taking again the example of CHD and serum cholesterol concentrations, although countries with a high dietary saturated fat intake are associated with higher average serum cholesterol levels this relationship cannot be extrapolated to individuals. Only a weak relationship exists between diet and serum cholesterol levels for individuals within societies with similar dietary patterns. It is suggested therefore that planning measures to reduce CHD through this risk factor would need to concentrate on population approaches to prevention, such as changing agricultural and national food policies (Nuffield Institute for Health, Centre for Health Economics and Royal College of Physicians, 1993).

Determining strategies

Although it seems rather obvious, one of the more important aspects of determining strategies for addressing healthcare problems is the identification of the particular agency and personnel to be charged with moving the programme forward. Linked to this is the question of who makes this decision. Much of the current discussion in the UK concerning the public health has occurred at the level of the Department of Health, which has published several documents and issued guidance to both purchasers and providers of healthcare services. Thus the requirements of *Working for Patients* (Department of Health, 1989b) decreed that District Health Authorities (DHAs) be responsible for assessing the health needs of their populations and arranging for those needs to be met. With specific respect to the public health function the Abraham report (Department of Health, 1993d) also identified the DHA and its Director of Public Health as responsible for providing a comprehensive public health strategy for their district. As noted earlier, these strategies are largely bounded by the targets set by *The Health of the Nation* (Department of Health, 1992a) and backed up and monitored by the information systems that this policy initiative has spawned, although it should be acknowledged that District Health Authorities are developing plans beyond this.

Although the white paper does provide both targets and strategies for meeting them, these latter have two characteristics that require further exploration. Firstly, strategies are almost exclusively focused at reducing risk factors, such as smoking and obesity, which are framed within both a biomedical and individualistic model of disease. Health, then, is conceptualised through a medical vision and responsibility for health is placed firmly with individuals. This individualistic model has been strongly criticised as denying the social aspect of health/illness; assuming that free choice exists to take steps towards a healthy lifestyle; and assuming that changes in knowledge lead to changes in behaviour (Naidoo, 1986). Risk, prevention and the individual are also discussed in Chapter 6.

Secondly, since little cognisance is given to the socio-economic causes which may underlie ill health, problems and their possible remedies remain within the biological domain. As Farrant and Russell (1985, p. 14) note the 'alternative model of CHD aetiology (i.e. that rooted in social factors such as poor nutrition and poverty) ultimately challenges orthodox medical practice by locating the point of intervention within the social and economic environment'. This would present certain territorial challenges to those professionals employed in this area. The field of health promotion (for this is ultimately largely what this argument centres on) is strongly contested among many professional groups, including nurses, doctors, social workers and educators. The role that these different professional groups may play in shaping the planning strategies that may be suggested, or indeed funded and adopted, cannot be ignored.

A fundamental challenge in planning is in deciding at what level the problem is to be tackled. Valenis (1992) describes a 'problem hierarchy' whereby it becomes apparent that each cause is a problem with its own causes. Suppose that, as a health visitor, you decide, after examining some comparative health statistics, that the rate of dental caries in your area is higher than average. What are the causes of this and what plans could you make to change the situation? A literature search might suggest that the rate of dental caries increases with decreasing public knowledge concerning the adverse effects of sweetened baby foods. This lack of knowledge among the public is then the problem, and this may have its own causes – perhaps funds have been cut back in this area so there are fewer personnel to provide information, or perhaps the local radio station now charges to broadcast health messages. This is examining the problem at a local and individual level. However, you might take a more global perspective and suggest that it is not a lack of knowledge concerning the danger of sweetened foods that is the cause of the problem, but the inability of families to pay for the more expensive foods that do not contain so much sugar. The cause of the problem then becomes low wages, or more fundamentally an inequality in the distribution of wealth. Thus each 'cause' has its own 'problem', and the key to effective planning is in determining how, when and by what means these could be most effectively tackled with the available resources.

Resources and target groups

Two other steps in the planning process – determining resources and determining target groups – remain to be discussed. The determination of whether sufficient and sustainable resources are available to take forward any new or modified service is obviously a crucial element in any planning exercise. Yet the numerous examples of both small and large projects which seem to founder on this very point indicate that strategic planning, in the health service at least, is far from the sophisticated exercise that those of us outside the enterprise are led to believe. New hospital buildings which cannot open for lack of resources; computer equipment that cannot fulfil the task for which it was envisaged (by the planners, perhaps, but probably not by the users); government telephone information lines which are unnecessary: the list is endless. Inefficient planning cannot be condemned in the light of unforeseen circumstances, but perhaps some of the disquiet raised in Chapter 4 concerning the problems of forecasting future trends in population statistics needs to be noted. The economic aspects of planning are, however, too wide a subject to tackle any further here; any further information may be obtained from the general texts suggested at the beginning of the chapter.

The question of determining which groups to target is again a logical step in any strategic planning exercise. It makes economic and organisational sense to target what are always limited resources towards those who will reap most benefit from them. Sometimes the target group for an intervention will form an easily recognisable population, e.g. pre-school children within the larger population of a district. Where a more selected group is required the epidemiological literature will usually provide information concerning the characteristics of those individuals who are particularly susceptible to certain conditions. These then become the target groups, and plans may be devised in order to arrange services to best meet the requirements of these people. Part of this exercise might include frequency counts of the target population and the way it is distributed in particular areas. Much conventional public health work and its associated epidemiology follows such paths. However, there are some very real dangers to this approach, which must be set in context against the essentially pragmatic requirements of a planning exercise.

Problems associated with targeting

Throughout, this book has striven to present epidemiology as an effective discipline which could provide many opportunities to nurses who wish to adapt its methods for the benefits of their own practice and the welfare of their clients. However, on several occasions along the way (see particularly Chapters 3 and 6) we have noted that the culture of conventional medical epidemiology may be at variance with the philosophy and ideology of nursing. An epidemiologically informed nursing will be able to challenge these dominant medical models, and yet retain concepts which may be useful to a more holistic interpretation of the discipline and its practice. The delineation of target groups for the purpose of planning services provides yet another example of where nursing, through a more flexible and eclectic approach, may provide insights beyond the biomedical.

The crucial question concerning the identification of groups who will be the target of services is: who is doing the identification? The paragraph above illustrates how it is all too easy to frame this question through the conventional epidemiological literature, which, using the methods of positivistic science, has associated certain factors with certain diseases, e.g. high blood pressure and strokes. The difficulty arises when the same information is used to define certain types of people as being more or less likely to develop certain conditions. There are two issues here that need addressing: firstly, the superimposition of the culture-bound disease categories of biomedicine to specific points in what is probably a wide biological continuum of physiological parameters, and secondly the use of apparently neutral scientific categories to depict certain groups as more vulnerable to particular conditions.

Disease categories and the biological data included within them are organised in different ways by different cultures (see also Chapter 2). Biomedicine is no exception to this, but as it has increased the depth of its biological understanding, the cultural component of biomedical disease classifications has become obscured. Biomedicine is just one particular framework for interpreting biological data. Biological measurements can be made in any individual in any culture, but the interpretation of the data is culturally mediated. Take the example of anaemia. In the 1960s epidemiological surveys revealed high levels of 'anaemia' in American black populations. Causes for this were considered to lie in the poor diet of these people, which was low in iron and high in starch. However, later anthropological research revealed that haemoglobin levels for black people, even those who were well nourished, were always lower than the equivalent white population (Garn, *et al.* 1981). This illustrates the crucial importance of distinguishing between biological data and biomedical categories of disease. Failure to recognise the biological differences in normal haemoglobin between the two populations and the application of a Western cultural category on these data would have labelled a large percentage of the normal black population as anaemic. This has obvious implications for the planning of services, for in this case resources would have been wasted in targeting a group who were not in fact in need of any intervention.

The second aspect of targeting that a more anthropological analysis reveals is the problem of the way in which epidemiology and much public health medicine conceptualises society or indeed culture. Chapters 1 and 6 describe how epidemiological studies explore risk factors for developing conditions, and attempt to identify groups who may display these factors. For example, Valenis (1992), in discussing cervical cancer and pap screening, suggests that those who are at high risk of the disease may be characterised by low income, multiple sexual partners, multiple pregnancies and low educational attainment.

Social and cultural factors have been increasingly included in epidemiological studies seeking to elucidate the aetiology and risk factors associated with the genesis of certain diseases. On a general front this is a welcome development and a recognition within epidemiology that social conditions may play a considerable role in disease aetiology. Nevertheless this has not led to a reconceptualisation of disease categories based on social origins, but rather a futile attempt to consign social and cultural aspects of sickness into discrete variables. Epidemiology has difficulties in conceptualising sociocultural factors, which cannot easily be reduced to such unitary variables. As Williams and Popay (1994b, pp. 102–3) note, 'If stress is equated to a simple life event score, class with occupation and diet with the type of fat used on bread, it is scarcely surprising that a large proportion of variance is unexplained'. The problem arises, therefore, through the particular conceptualisations that biomedical researchers use in this context. At the core of this argument is the problematic way in which public health researchers use the concepts of culture and society as an explanatory variable in their analyses. The construction of epidemiological categories that portray groups at risk of AIDs will be used to illustrate this point.

Glick Schiller (1992) discusses how, in AIDS research in the USA, health researchers and anthropologists hold differing models of the mechanisms through which behaviour that puts individuals at risk for AIDS is affected by the wider socio-economic context in which they live. For the biomedical health workers, certain minority populations are at risk because they are members of cultures which deviate in lifestyles and mores from the general population. In other words, risky behaviour emanates from culture. The concept of the 'at risk group' promulgated by epidemiology thereby legitimises the attribution of lethal diseases such as AIDS to culturally different groups.

In contrast, anthropologists contend that risky behaviour is not a product of any particular culture, say Hispanic or black, but is embedded in the interaction of those cultures with broader economic conditions and power relationships. Thus the public health approach to HIV has 'presented risk for AIDS as linked to culturally distinct populations rather than to specific behaviours that increase the possibility of infection' (Glick Schiller, 1992, p. 245). In this way, risk becomes embedded in identity rather than action. This racial and ethnic categorisation of risky behaviour may be highly misleading and result in the formulation of health plans that both have no basis in reality and furthermore act to stigmatise certain groups in society.

At the heart of this lies some of the problems with attempting to draw boundaries around populations and designate them as at risk – a favourite occupation of epidemiologists. For as Stone (1990, pp. 91–2) notes 'risk factors and designations of high risk groups do not grow immediately out of epidemiological research. They are created in a social context which involves judgement, persuasion, bargaining and political manoeuvring... about what is considered a risk factor and how broadly categories are drawn'. The two examples above illustrate the extreme caution that is required in any planning exercise that delineates groups as 'at risk'. On the one hand, the practical exigencies of targeting resources may compel planners to utilise epidemiological information in this way, but the deeper ramifications of these categorisations must be recognised and acknowledged.

Planning which strategies should be employed to tackle health problems is thus more complex than outward appearances might dictate. Indeed, it has been suggested that, in the UK at least, although managers are skilled in determining current provision, and public health doctors are adept at assessing health needs, 'there is little science in either determining the best way to meet those needs or assessing the effectiveness of any interventions' (Harris and Shapiro, 1994). Two crucial points emerge from the discussion above:

1. The 'web of causation' is complex, and for many chronic conditions aetiology is both multifactorial and often incomplete. Selecting the most effective strategies to solve healthcare problems is not therefore a simple task of selecting individual packages or campaigns off the shelf in isolated attempts to tackle these problems. In many cases it must be realised that the research information on which rational decisions might be based is lacking.

2. Health strategies are socially constructed. Many perspectives exist, each being driven by interested parties. Thus different frameworks for conceptualising health problems and their potential solutions may exist. These are particularly relevant in the case of different professional groups who make use of different models of health, and also the government, which is pursuing its own agenda largely embedded in seeking efficiency and effectiveness of service with particular regard to cost. With regard to this, an unpublished survey of purchasing plans in London (quoted by Harris and Shapiro (1994)) notes that changes were concerned more with efficiency issues than with trying to provide more appropriate or effective care.

Any framework for planning services therefore exists both within the larger organisational context of the NHS and related services and within the wider milieu of the political economies of the day. It is a collage of often uncertain knowledge set against, and operationalised within, a particular sociocultural context.

The evaluation of strategies

Evaluation and audit

Whether one is planning for a new programme of health services or for modification of existing arrangements, it is essential that mechanisms for evaluation are included. Planning and evaluation form part of a cyclical process whereby plans are formulated and implemented, leading to changes in activity which continue for some time, after which an evaluation occurs. This in its turn will lead to modification in the original plans and a new cycle of planning/action/evaluation/ planning will occur. Figure 5.1 illustrates this cycle. Furthermore this process can be envisaged as a spiral which moves upwards towards the final solution of the original goals of the planning process. At the start of the planning spiral it is likely that information about the problem and the optimum strategy for addressing it will be limited. However, after several cycles have been completed more information will become available to the planner, who is then in a position to make more informed choices to refine the original strategy.

In some respects, evaluation may be seen as part of a more general concern with the standard of health services, which is also encompassed within quality assurance programmes and audit. Since 1984, when the concepts of general management became firmly established in the NHS, there has been an increasing emphasis on business principles and a 'managed approach to quality' has been encouraged by the Department of Health (Brooks, 1992). In addition, the *Health of the Nation* strategy has provoked a greater awareness of the need to demonstrate the benefits of any newly planned service. This initiative

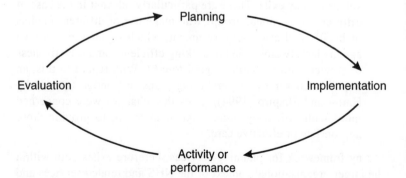

Figure 5.1 *The planning and evaluation cycle.*

is of course driven not only through an altruistic notion to provide the most effective and efficient services, but also by the political necessity to demonstrate the legitimacy of this particular governmental policy. This has led to the development of mechanisms through which progress towards the targets of the white paper can be measured. Thus national indicators to monitor progress towards the primary targets have been issued (Department of Health, 1993e), and new health surveys conducted (Department of Health, 1993f).

The concept of quality will be further explored in the following section in this chapter. It is mentioned here in order to clarify the differences and similarities between audit and evaluation.

In simple terms, **audit** is the systematic review of practice with the objective of improving it. The first stage involves defining a standard that should be achieved – for example, how soon after admission patients should meet their named nurses. The standard may be derived through consensus or from guidelines issued by experts or professional bodies. Following this, performance is assessed in relation to the agreed standard. The assessment should suggest ways in which practice may be modified to attain closer agreement with the standard. Finally, these changes must be agreed with practitioners and put into action to await a further cycle of audit.

The purpose of **evaluation** is to estimate how effectively the original aims determined during service planning are being met (McIver, 1991). In other words it is concerned with judging the value of strategies that have been put into place by the new plans. Service evaluation should occur at regular intervals and usually demands a wide range of information.

In many respects, therefore, evaluation and audit are similar activities. Evaluation matches up performance with the pre-stated objectives of a planning exercise, and audit matches up performance with a pre-stated standard of care. Both should produce recommendations, which should then lead to changes in the activities being scrutinised with the goal of more closely matching the original objectives. The difference between evaluation and planning most usually lies in the scale of the exercise. The evaluation of planning strategies is often a more global exercise, which may consider many aspects of the provision of a service. Not only is it to do with the effectiveness of a service, but also its efficiency. Efficiency being 'the ability of a healthcare intervention to produce the desired outcome in a defined population under ideal conditions' (Hopkins, 1993, p. 117). The use of resources, and what they might be used for if they were not being used for this service, is also often central to any evaluation. In contrast, audit may be quite local and is primarily concerned with effectiveness, where effectiveness is 'the extent to which an outcome is achieved under the usual conditions of care in "real life"' (Hopkins, 1993, p. 117). Although audit should allow a comparison with a preset standard, it may occur without any extensive preplanning as to the various options that might be adopted in any instance of service provision. Evaluation as part of planning has a strategic element which audit in some senses lacks. Nevertheless the two activities do have many commonalities.

The evaluation plan

In evaluating a new way of providing a service, therefore, a central question is whether the original aims and objectives envisaged during the planning of the change are being met, and if they will continue to be met in the future. Does it achieve what we thought it would? Is it cost effective? What is it like to nurse in this way? Do patients prefer it? How could we improve it? These are the types of question that need to be raised. An evaluation is necessary to answer such questions. The requisite information will cover a wide range of topics and will need to be collected from several sources if a meaningful evaluation is to be undertaken. Feedback from both the consumers and staff is required, together with any pertinent information that may be routinely collected during care.

The effectiveness of any particular nursing action depends on the eye of the beholder; for managers, cost efficiency may be paramount, whereas for the user comfort and convenience would be more important characteristics. A comprehensive evaluation should at least examine the following: access, choice, quality, benefits, economy and side effects. The following elements will need to be included in any evaluation:

- a plan of the programme and its **objectives** (if the service is already in existence and there is no plan then a reconstruction must be devised)
- the identification of instruments to measure whether the objectives have been met
- the formulation of data collection forms and schedules
- a plan for analysis
- a system for producing recommendations, feedback and implementation of suggested changes
- a timetable for each stage and for future evaluations.

The objectives of the planning programme should form the basis for the evaluation. Any new programme plan will have aims and objectives. **Aims** are generally conceived in broad terms and reflect the original nature of the health problem. For example, for an infection control nurse the aim of a new programme might be to reduce the rate of nosocomial urinary tract infections.

Objectives will relate to each stage of the problem hierarchy and specify the outcomes to be achieved. An objective is a specific, realistic and measurable statement of the change that it is hoped a particular plan will achieve. Objectives are SMART – Specific, Measurable, Agreed, Realistic and Timetabled. Continuing the same example, an objective for the infection control nurse's plan might be 'to stop the use of urethral catheters in nursing home patients who are incontinent'. The objective would then need a time period by which this should be achieved, and a mechanism for its accomplishment (i.e. another objective). This latter might be a series of seminars for nurses who work in residential homes. Just as the problem hierarchy reveals that each cause is a problem with its own causes, so each objective reveals secondary objectives in this way. For each programme objective a method of evaluation will need to be devised.

Two cardinal principles should guide the **collection of data**. Firstly, the information that is obtained must be *accurate*. In this respect it is necessary to use data collecting instruments that have a high validity rating, i.e. they actually record the attribute that is of interest. Secondly, the information must be *useful*, in other words it must relate to issues that the providers and recipients of the care consider important. Thus it is necessary to obtain valid data that reflect the experiences and opinions of all those involved, and to ensure that this information can be used to answer the questions that prompted the evaluation in the first place.

The particular emphasis of the evaluation is also critical. Asking patients about the *process* of undergoing a particular procedure is different from enquiring about the *outcome* of that care. Similarly, another way of approaching the evaluation is to ask clients about the service that they *need*. People's opinion of nursing care may not be directly reconcilable with their views on the care that they would like in an ideal world – allowance is made for the provider 'doing the best which they can'.

Accurate information may not be useful information. It is crucial therefore that any evaluation that is undertaken has a clear set of pre-stated aims. Different information will be required to answer the various questions that may arise from any particular perspective.

Each objective of the plan that is addressed in the evaluation will need to be measured and included in the analysis. Both quantitative and qualitative measures may be produced. However, health economists and planners are more likely to give credence only to the former. Thus statistical information is widely used in this type of exercise. So the infection control nurse could conduct a prevalence survey of catheter usage in incontinent patients before and after the introduction of her plan to determine how far her educational activities had influenced practice.

Needless to say, this quantitative type of evaluation would only provide information concerning the extent to which the plan's objectives had been met. If a programme is meeting its objectives within acceptable criteria, then if resource allocation remains the same it will probably continue in the same format. If there had been no reduction in catheter usage, although the nurse would know that the objective of the plan had not been met she would not know why. Other more qualitative strategies, for example interviewing nurses or observing them in their everyday work, would be required to determine why they still continued to catheterise patients who were incontinent. This type of information will be more valuable during the phase of the evaluation concerned with determining how the plan will need to be **modified**, **fed back** and **reimplemented** to start another cycle in the planning spiral.

Evaluations may also reveal unforeseen factors, which may be contributing to the original problem. The evaluation report will need to consider whether any actions need to be instituted as a result of these revelations. The findings of the evaluation may also point to the need for further more extensive epidemiological studies to elucidate the situation further. The evaluation of new or existing plans for the provision of healthcare services is essential. Not only does an evaluation determine whether the original aims and objectives of the plan are being met, it demonstrates to what extent this is occurring, and it may also reveal other aspects of the process of care that were not apparent at the outset.

Covert aspects of evaluation

At one level the evaluation of a plan is a practical exercise to determine the value of the activities subsumed within it. But from another perspective, evaluations, just like anything else in life, may carry some covert aspects that are not visible given a cursory scrutiny. This is particularly important with regard to the setting of quantitative limits on objectives. For example, the infection control nurse in our example needed at the outset of the plan to set a limit on her objective of reducing the use of catheters. If, instead of stating that she wished catheter usage for incontinence to cease altogether a 50% reduction would be acceptable, then the chances of achieving this latter target would be much greater.

Dangers may arise, then, when the quantification of the effectiveness of the programme lies within the control of the planner. If an underestimate is made of the ability of a new plan to tackle a problem, then the resulting evaluation may appear quite impressive. As Valenis (1992, p. 422) notes, 'The smart planner will choose an intermediate to low estimate. Too high or too much of an overestimate could make a program look pretty bad'. This emphasises the need to scrutinise carefully the original premises upon which the evaluation of new plans are based.

Another aspect of evaluation which is related to the ethos of the new public health is described by Ashton and Seymour (1991). If public health is to be truly community-centred, then not only must people define their own health problems, but they must also be 'central to any assessment of whether an intervention is worthwhile' (Ashton and Seymour, 1991, p. 110). This returns to the point made above concerning the usefulness of any information collected during an evaluation, and how different people will have different perspectives upon what is useful. If planning for public health is to take the spirit of the Ottawa Charter (World Health Organisation, 1986) as its framework, then serious consideration must be given as to how evaluation may become more focused on the priorities of ordinary people.

The requirement for positive indicators of health and ways of describing concepts such as empowerment, networking and community morale must therefore be developed to replace the existing quantitative pathological measures of 'health'. In addition, the context or environment (see above) that surrounds the way in which people are able to act to take healthy choices must be considered. These factors have a significant influence on the success that any new health plan can hope to achieve. Finally, although it must be acknowledged that traditional epidemiological evaluations, with their currently strong emphasis on value for money, are undoubtedly necessary, more community-initiated and conducted research is required (see, for example, Wainwright, 1993).

The first section of this chapter has reviewed the planning of health services in general and the planning of public health services in particular, since this is an area where traditionally epidemiology has played a prominent role. The discussion has centred on the pragmatic aspects of planning by addressing three questions:

- How should the healthcare 'problems' of a population be identified?

- How should services be arranged to address these problems?
- How should the chosen services be evaluated?

Emphasis has been given to a conventional framework through which much planning historically has been, and continues to be, set. Despite this, several more controversial points have been raised which are concerned principally with the issue of who sets agendas. As we have seen, this may have a considerable influence upon those phenomena that are considered problems, the type of healthcare strategies which may be adopted, and the mechanisms through which they are evaluated. The planning of services often rests in the hands of powerful professional groups or the government, who have certain vested interests beyond providing the most effective and efficient services. These 'interests' may operate openly, as is being increasingly observed in the internal market, where different providers vie for health business. Alternatively, they may act at a covert level submerged within the historical practices and ideologies of the health service, hidden even from those who are involved in their pursuit. The tendency to shore up the tradition of professional territorialism dies hard, but may go almost unnoticed by those steeped in its culture, who continue to fashion their planning of public health activities around the framework of biologically oriented hospital medicine.

IS RATIONAL PLANNING POSSIBLE?

Thus far this chapter has provided a conventional (well almost!) account of planning for one particular service – the public health function – and what could be more straightforward than the steps of the exercise as outlined above? Indeed, the solidity of this practical procedure defies any spontaneous questioning of its foundations. However, the second section of this chapter will challenge the basis of much of what has been discussed above by posing the question of whether, given the present organisation of the NHS, rational planning is possible. The arguments that will be developed are based on the premise that, although the cardinal principles of the NHS ('first that it should be available to all people, and second that it covers all necessary forms of health care' (Ministry of Health, 1944, p. 9)) are continually reiterated and used as a defence against changes, the practical and philosophical bases of these principles remain unclear. As Seedhouse (1994, p. vii) remarks, 'the principles have become an unquestioned, unexamined, article of faith'.

What, it may be asked, has this to do with epidemiology, planning or indeed nursing? Firstly, through the activities of planning, epidemiology is involved in the determination of much of what is ideologically embodied in the ethos of the 1944 white paper. In particular, as discussed above, epidemiology frequently provides the information that allows an estimation of health needs and how they should best be met in an equitable and effective fashion. Thus epidemiology impinges, albeit indirectly, upon strategies concerned with the determination of the nature, range, quality and quantity of services. Any analysis of planning, and epidemiology's role within it, must therefore devolve from a clear understanding of what is meant by such terms as health need, health gain and quality. If these concepts are not clarified, then planning becomes an inconsistent and irrational activity floating in a sea of changing targets. Fundamentally this reduces to the question of whether the major organisation in the UK providing healthcare services – the NHS – has a clear purpose (as supposedly enshrined in the above principles). While the purpose of the NHS remains undefined, planning remains in limbo, bereft of any fundamental basic vision on which to rest its central aims and objectives. In other words, if we do not know what we are aiming for, then planning the way there will be a tricky and largely fruitless exercise.

At first glance, nursing's role in attempts to untangle these largely philosophical considerations might appear to be rather small. Certainly nursing has not in the past involved itself greatly in any debates about the fundamental basis of healthcare provision. However, in contrast with medicine, nursing has a far more eclectic and all-embracing ideology of health and its correlates in illness and disease. For many doctors the health service has until relatively recently been solely regarded as a *medical service*. Any broader conceptualisation of health embedded within wider sociocultural and political contexts has not been countenanced by a profession deeply ingrained in the biomedical model of disease. However, any cogent re-evaluation of principles such as health need and health gain must embrace this wider conceptualisation. Nursing, with its long-established holistic ideology, will not only be more receptive to any radical questioning and reworking of these taken for granted principles, but may also be in a position to lead the way with analysing and implementing the new ideas associated with them.

The crucial importance of challenging the conventional approach to planning is highlighted by recent documents from the NHS Management Executive District Health Authority project. Discussing health needs assessment, this report proposes a dual approach derived from an epidemiological/economic standpoint and 'a pragmatic approach blurring the distinction between need and demand, science and opinion' (NHSME, 1991, p. 3). Williams and Popay (1994b, p. 101) criticise this dichotomy of methodology as reproducing 'the conventional distinction between the scientific and the non scientific, between issues of objective need and clinical quality on the one hand and matters of opinion or preference and non clinical quality issues on the other'. It is the responsibility of nurses and other social scientists to expose the limitations of these classical models and suggest more appropriate approaches to research in this area.

The original statements about the purpose of the NHS as delineated in the white paper (Ministry of Health, 1944) crystallise into four simple principles – need, quality, equality and cost. The remainder of this chapter will be devoted to examining just two of these which are particularly pertinent to epidemiology – need and quality.

Challenging the concept of need

Need and planning

Healthcare planners have long aspired to the idea that healthcare provision might be based on prior assessment of health needs. Similarly, in the field of epidemiology considerable time has been spent in striving to define what was encompassed by the concept of need, on the basis that this should form the rationale through which planning could be structured. Several definitions have been produced, among them the proposal that **perceived health needs** occur when 'an individual or his family identify and acknowledge an "abnormality"', **unperceived needs** being conditions unrecognised by the aforementioned, but 'potentially discoverable by a practitioner' (Alderson, 1976, p. 29). However, for as long as some epidemiologists have been attempting to clarify the definition of need, there have been others who regard this concept as useless. For example, Glass (1976, p. 43), commenting on Alderson's definition, suggests that '"need" is too ill-defined a concept to be of practical use in considering the deployment of medical resources'. In the same paper the idea is raised that because 'need' might be measurable, and is called 'need', there is a notion that the 'need' ought to be met.

Working for Patients (Department of Health, 1989b) clearly defined the requirement for district health authorities to be responsible for assessing the health needs of their populations and arranging for these health needs to be met. Similarly, hospitals were charged with providing efficient and effective health services to meet the needs identified by health authorities. Needs assessment has thereby become a 'growth industry' within the health service as managers strive to meet this particular planning objective. However, if the philosophical basis underlying the question 'What is a need?' is not properly addressed at the outset, then practical needs assessment will lack the theoretical underpinning essential to its operationalisation. What is required is a reasoned and specific definition of need.

Definitions of need

Seedhouse (1994, p. 28) suggests that there are currently at least three different versions of 'need' used in the NHS:

'1. Health care need is the ability to benefit from healthcare (Stevens and Gabbay, 1991).
2. Health care need exists when there is ill health (Liss, 1990).
3. Health care need is a matter of expert judgement (Liss, 1990).'

All of these definitions can be challenged through a philosophical analysis (Seedhouse, 1994). If need is defined as *the ability to benefit from healthcare* then the only condition for there being a healthcare need is the existence of appropriate services to meet it. The logical expansion of this is that if there is no healthcare service to meet a need then a person cannot be *in need*. Likewise, as healthcare services increase so will need, and it would be impossible to reduce needs by providing more services.

If need is only manifest in *the presence of ill health*, then a highly restricted notion of health as the absence of disease is brought to bear. By this definition only those cases of ill health as defined by the health service (i.e. within the auspices of medicine) are in need. As with the first definition, this interpretation neatly confines the analysis of need to a medically oriented and dominated health service. It implies that health need can be defined only through the limits and extent of the NHS, clearly an erroneous conclusion.

The third definition, that expert judgement should be the avenue through which needs are defined (the normative definition), is a common interpretation in the present health service system. It assumes that not only are experts able to assess needs, but also to decide what these needs are to start with. The problems with this stem not only from the familiar arguments concerning who has the right to judge the health needs of individuals, but also from the historical organisation of the NHS. This latter ensures that the assessors are experts only in a narrowly defined ill health which is consonant with medical services and medical knowledge. Thus the *status quo* within the health service is maintained.

The discussion above illustrates that, far from being an objective concept, free from ideology, needs are defined and used in a variety of ways within current health service planning. What is more, these conceptualisations of need are used in assessment exercises which provide the criterion for rationing healthcare, and yet the vagueness of this procedure is not revealed. If a number of different ways to assess need coexist, none of which has any clear philosophical reasoning behind it, then the inconsistency of the entire procedure should be made more explicit.

A more insightful analysis of the nature of need would assist in clarifying this health service principle in order that it may be used in a more meaningful way, for there is no doubt that the assessment of health needs is an extremely important activity. However, the muddles that currently surround need as it is used in the NHS obscure its usefulness. Adding to this, Frankel (1991, p. 1588) purports that need has two distinct meanings as 'circumstances in which a thing/course of action is required; [and] a lack of necessaries, poverty'. He also suggests that a conflation between the needs of populations and the need for specific interventions has occurred, adding to the semantic confusion in this area. The foregoing makes it clear therefore that defining need in the abstract is far from easy, and this in itself has led to the problems with defining health needs in practice. A more perceptive analysis of the philosophical basis of need, such as is provided by Seedhouse (1994), may assist in clearing a way through this conceptual jungle.

Philosophical approaches to need

Two definitions commonly discussed within philosophy include the conceptualisation of needs as **the difference between two states** (Liss, 1990), and the view that need is an **exceptional category** (Thomson, 1987). This latter purports that some needs, such as shelter, food and medicine, are fundamental and from a moral standpoint should be met. These needs are not needed for something else, a prior purpose, but are essentials without which disastrous harm develops. They are intrinsic to our very well being and stand alone. In contrast, as a difference between an actual state and a goal, needs may be conceptualised as neither fundamental nor as physical things. Need is simply the difference between the actual state and the desired state (Liss, 1990). For example, if no facilities exist to provide for the delivery of babies at home and a woman's goal is to have a home birth, then there can be said to be a need to fill this gap. The need is neither fundamental nor a physical thing, but a means to reach a desired end.

The contention that some needs are fundamental can always be challenged. Even something as fundamental as food may in certain circumstances not be needed. Where, for example, a political protester is on hunger strike to meet political objectives or needs, then food is not required. In fact, the protestor's need is for no food. However, if needs are conceived as instrumental to achieving an objective state they may vary according to people's viewpoints or circumstances, and are not fixed and immutable, nor linked to moral categories. For Seedhouse (1994) the idea of needs as instrumental is both logical and important, since it does not presuppose the limits of need, as need is dependent upon purpose. This he contends underlines the crucial necessity of disentangling what the purpose of the health service is, for the assessment of needs is inextricably linked with this. Needs are thereby assessed not according to whether they are fundamental or not, but in line with the extent to which providing them makes certain things possible.

A further point should be made regarding the contention that non-reasoned needs (e.g. hunger) should take precedence over reasoned needs (wants), such as the desire to own a Mercedes car, for in the majority of cases it is very problematic to distinguish clearly between these two categories of needs and wants. Furthermore, capitulating to the argument that non-reasoned 'needs' are somehow more basic than reasoned 'wants' leads to the situation where biological (or unconscious) needs are perceived as more important than reasoned wants. Action to meet these biological needs, in other words medical action, then takes precedence over other actions. This reasoning is consonant with the medical model of health, the present functioning of the NHS and the 'category mistake that disease and health are on a single continuum' (Seedhouse, 1994, p. 38).

Needs assessment – a critical approach

The discussion above has attempted to illustrate some of the problems surrounding the concept of need, and therefore some of the difficulties that are associated with the uncritical use of this principle to guide health service planning. It is apparent that in current usage need has several definitions, and various perspectives from which it can be viewed. None of the three definitions proposed at the beginning of the section is problem-free, and all are too weak to determine consistent policy-making. Need for healthcare cannot be defined purely on the premise of existing services, or through the opinion of experts. Nor can health needs be exclusively bounded by the parameters of clinical medicine. Health in the wider world is not solely associated with disease or clinical priorities. Nursing with its more holistic paradigm of health and illness has long recognised this.

A more perspicacious conceptualisation of need is required if planning is to have any basis in the realities of what ordinary people require for health. From this position, the instrumental account of need appears promising, since it 'requires the clearest specification of purpose, demands that potential benefits can be demonstrated, and allows subjects to be involved in needs assessment.' (Seedhouse, 1994, p. 42). If this definition is used as a framework, health needs assessment will come some way towards determining 'real' needs rather than needs as perceived by those working in the health services or government, these latter needs being purely restricted to what the NHS can supply. If these restrictions are not lifted, then needs assessment surveys will be little more than self-fulfilling prophecies which must inevitably reinforce the organisational fortress that the NHS has become.

The importance of expanding the model of health needs beyond the fortifications of the NHS is well illustrated by the framework that underlies **popular epidemiology** (see Chapters 1 and 2). This pursuit of epidemiological knowledge by lay people has arisen through their dissatisfaction with the explanations provided by the conventional scientific community. Popular epidemiology has been fuelled mostly by environmental concerns and often by particular incidents where governmental responses or public enquiries have failed to satisfy ordinary citizens. Many instances exist in the USA – one example is the refusal of the residents of Woburn, Massachusetts, to accept the conclusion of the experts from the Centers for Disease Control that the increased incidence of childhood leukaemia in the town was not attributable to the water supply (see Brown (1987, 1992) for a full description of this case). In the UK, the contamination of the water supply in Camelford, Cornwall, in July 1988 precipitated the emergence of the locally organised Camelford Scientific Advisory Panel, which undertook its own investigation independent from the governmental enquiry led by Dame Barbara Clayton (Cornwall and the Isles of Scilly District Health Authority, 1989; Department of Health, 1991b). An account of this incident and the part that local people played in gathering and analysing epidemiological data may be found in Williams and Popay (1994a).

Popular epidemiology provides another instance therefore which illustrates that health, and therefore health need, cannot be conceptualised solely through a biomedical framework. The health needs of the people of Woburn and Camelford were clearly at variance with those which official bodies were proposing. Health for these people, as for all of us, cannot simply be constructed through a narrative of biological dysfunctions which can be met through biomedical interventions provided by the current structural organisation of the NHS. The health needs of these people were clearly 'real' – were they being recognised?

The official Clayton report stated that 'In our view it is not possible to attribute the very real current health complaints to the toxic effects of the incident, except in as much as they are the consequence of the sustained anxiety naturally felt by many people' (Cornwall and the Isles of Scilly District Health Authority, 1989, p. 14). Thus not only are these health problems denied a 'biological' aetiology, but they are also relegated to a community diagnosis of 'sustained anxiety'. This latter explanation of the community's beliefs 'was a way of indicating its unreliability and, therefore its distance from the standards of scientific discourse' (Williams and Popay, 1994a, p. 132). Any thoughtful analysis of health needs must go beyond this type of rigid reasoning and embrace a more holistic definition of health and the meaning which it has in the everyday world.

Another approach to health needs assessment is put forward by Ong and Humphris (1994), who contend that purchasers and providers must pool their expertise and work alongside the community. Suggesting that users should jointly participate in the definition of need, the identification of priorities and evaluation, these authors point out that this approach will require a 'paradigm ·shift whereby the community perspective will become the guiding principle for setting priorities in healthcare' (Ong and Humphris, 1994, p. 80).

This multidisciplinary approach is epitomised by rapid appraisal, a method which attempts to bring together the perspectives of communities through a dialogue with decision-makers. It is characterised by two objectives – continuity and commitment to the community, and action through the delivery of results (Rifkin, 1992). The use of rapid appraisal in the UK is discussed by Annett and Rifkin (1990), and several projects are outlined by Ong and Humphris (1994). Central to rapid appraisal are in-depth qualitative interviews with key informants in the community in order to identify needs. This information is analysed alongside other sources of qualitative and quantitative data obtained through geographical mapping, observation, census and epidemiological techniques. Particular insights have been gained through the comparison of community and professional priorities, which in many of the projects have differed. More alarmingly, significant differences were noted between professionals' perceptions of what the community told them they wanted and the actual community view. This raises serious questions about the ability of professionals to elicit or interpret community views, and underlines the compelling cultural forces that covertly or overtly shape the way different groups within society act.

A question of quality

Quality and the NHS

Over the last ten years a 'culture of quality', or at least an assumed 'culture of quality', has come to dominate almost every encounter in the NHS. From quality circles, quality assurance, audit and evaluation to total quality management, every professional group and every consumer of healthcare has been enmeshed in this ethos. A cursory glance at any of the journals devoted to health service issues demonstrates the almost obsessive hold that this idea now has, especially in the minds of government and local hospital management. The drive for quality has been influenced in particular ways by *Working for Patients* (Department of Health, 1989b), which stresses the need to quickly address quality in those aspects of the service that the public sees as most lacking. Specifically, these include appointment systems, information for patients and reception arrangements. Thus purchasers have been charged with developing comprehensive quality assurance programmes while paying particular attention to the above items.

The UK has no official body with overall responsibility for assuring quality in healthcare, although the Audit Commission was given specific briefs under *Working for Patients* (Department of Health, 1989b) to pursue one-off inquiries. This lack of an overall agency has enabled the various healthcare professions to retain much of the responsibility for quality assurance.

Given the above it is not surprising that for the planners of health services quality has become a watchword, ignored at their peril. Quality has been invoked to embrace the idea articulated alongside the four principles of the NHS that not only should healthcare services be comprehensive, but that the 'best services' should be provided (Ministry of Health, 1944). Thus in the language of the NHS 'best services' have become synonymous with 'quality services'. However, as with the concept of need there is no clear understanding of what exactly is meant by 'quality' when it is applied to the provision of health services. Once again, therefore, conceptual muddles obfuscate one of the central principles on which the planning of health services hinge.

One of the most widely used definitions of quality in healthcare (Maxwell *et al.*, 1983) contends that the following elements should all be included: appropriateness, equity, accessibility, effectiveness, acceptability and efficiency. Although this definition appears at first sight to be both meaningful and comprehensive, a little scraping at the surface reveals its transparency and incompleteness. Take equity: if services are to be fairly shared among the population who need them (which is what Maxwell *et al.* suggest), then this immediately begs several crucial questions. Which services? Which population? What is a fair share? Similar criticisms may be levelled at all the remaining elements that are suggested to define quality.

There is little to be gained by defining quality in relation to other terms, such as equity or appropriateness, for which the NHS holds no clear definition either. Furthermore, in practice the elements of the definition may easily be working against each other. How then can they be contained within the same definition? For example, in the interests of efficiency many of the London teaching hospitals have been twinned up. However, the amalgamation of particular departments and their location at one site may reduce accessibility for the consumers of the service. It is clear that, as with the concept of need, some considerable groundwork is necessary before any meaningful definition of quality as applied to the health service can emerge. Without this basic questioning of what these terms really mean, and an analysis of how they are currently used, then any plans to ensure the quality of services will be flawed at the outset.

A business ethos

Stemming from the first restructuring of the NHS early in the 1970s (Department of Health and Social Security, 1972) through the Griffiths reorganisation (Department of Health and Social Security, 1983), and culminating in the creation of the internal market in the late 1980s, a new management ethos modelled on modern business lines entered the world of healthcare provision. Integral to this has been the introduction of commercial ideas and their associated practice and language. In this the NHS has been much influenced by the USA, where health systems analysis is a major activity. Under this aegis, quality assurance has been strongly advocated and numerous staff have been appointed to take this initiative further within the NHS. Many of these new appointments have been filled by nurse managers displaced during the Griffiths reorganisation. Two important points therefore emerge. Firstly, many of the ideas about quality in the NHS are being borrowed from the world of commerce, and secondly the responsibility for assuring quality falls in a number of different camps. As Ranade suggests (1994, p. 105), 'early evidence of the implementation of audit and the battery of other quality initiatives in the NHS suggest that doctors, nurses, managers and other staff not to mention consumers, still step delicately in a ritual dance which recognises established prerogatives and power'. This latter point will be addressed below (in *Whose quality?*), while the problems associated with importing quality concepts from business will be tackled here.

In the business world several definitions of quality exist. Two that have been adopted for use in healthcare provision will be discussed:

- The British Standard definition (Oakland, 1989, p. 3), which states that quality is 'the totality of features and characteristics of a product or a service that bear on its ability to satisfy stated or implied needs'.
- The fit for purpose definition, which states that 'if the product is fit for the intended purpose then it is quality' (Seedhouse, 1994, p. 49).

The first of these definitions makes the fundamental error of confusing quality with qualities. In general parlance something is said to be 'of quality' if it provides something above average – an excellent service etc. Belgian chocolates are quality chocolates: they are distinguishable and preferable to those bought in the local market at a cut price just before Christmas. A diagnostic service which provides immediate testing and the provision of results within 24 hours might be said to be a quality service.

However, the British standard definition equates quality with attributes and characteristics, i.e. with qualities. Every service will have certain characteristics, which may or may not be of quality. Take the example of a practice nurse who decides to set up a special clinic to advise clients who are going abroad for their holidays. Those on the GP's list may regard this as a valuable addition to the range of services offered in their local health centre – it is a desirable attribute, a good quality. However, if the nurse running the clinic was unclear about which vaccinations were required for which countries then one could not say this was a service of quality. This definition fails, therefore, since it does not explain what quality is. Furthermore, if quality is dependent upon satisfying needs, then a question must be raised as to whose need, and whether this need might change with time, place and person. This last point will be discussed further below, but it is mentioned here to illustrate the ambiguity and lack of clarity that are inherent in this definition.

The 'fitness for purpose definition' of quality is widely used within the health service. However, as with the analysis of needs discussed in the previous section, this definition is meaningless in the absence of any clear statement of the purpose that the service is said to be fit for. Under this definition any service could be considered a quality service as long as it had a purpose. This might be acceptable in business, but in the world of healthcare other conjunctures apply. So a new plan which set out to remove all people over the age of 85 years from GP's lists could, if it achieved its aim, be said to provide a quality service. This is patent nonsense. What makes this version of quality so attractive to health service planners, however, is its intrinsic and sinister ability to fit into the existing *status quo*. With the ultimate purpose of the NHS far from clear, quality becomes defined according to what is available, since this is the only way in which purpose is currently conceptualised in the NHS (see also the discussion of needs assessment above).

The problems associated with attempting to transfer jargon and concepts between these two totally different worlds, that of healthcare and that of commerce, are all too apparent therefore. Definitions culled from business imply that quality is relative; that is, quality is not intrinsic to a service or thing, but depends on the circumstances which surround it. Conceived in this way, quality, rather like some fictional character from *Star Trek*, is an ever-changing phenomenon. In an NHS which lacks a coherent purpose and which is therefore increasingly guided by politics and lately the internal market, the adoption of 'commercial quality' is both conceptually naïve, and ultimately of scant value in building a genuine health service.

Whose quality?

It has been assumed that quality is an essential element to devising strategic healthcare plans in the 1990s. However, the discussion thus far has made it clear that not only is the definition of quality in severe disarray, but quality frequently lies in the eye of the beholder. Thus a constant theme runs through this area concerning who is defining quality, and by what standards this exercise is proceeding. The answers to these questions feed not only into the conceptual difficulties discussed above, but also more pragmatic organisational issues.

Taking this latter point, Politt (1992) has argued that responsibility for quality in the NHS is divided along tribal lines which reflect the boundaries of professional territories and the struggles for power that occur around these. The determination of quality may proceed by quite different routes according to the arena in which it is pursued. Thus medical audit, until very recently, was very much a private activity carried out within the profession and protected from public scrutiny, although with the recent publication of league tables for waiting lists and post-operative mortality in UK hospitals some of this secrecy has been removed, as performance tables become available not only to purchasers of services, but also to the public. In contrast, nursing audit has always been a relatively open activity largely in the control of managers. As a result it illustrates particularly well the conflicts that may occur through the different perceptions that various groups may have on 'quality care'. For practitioners individualised care as exemplified by primary nursing and the concept of the named nurse has come to be the hallmark of quality nursing. In contrast, managerial strategies for assessing workload (such as Criteria for Care) utilise estimations of patient dependency. This has led to an increasingly transient workforce which is deployed as and when it is needed (Procter, 1990). In these circumstances continuity – essential to individualised care – is difficult to maintain. Two very different perspectives on quality, one aspired to by management and the other by practitioners, thereby emerge.

This returns us to the conceptual difficulties surrounding the definition of quality, for the British Standard definition stated that quality had something to do with the 'ability to satisfy stated or implied needs'. Applying this in the NHS, such needs may relate either to the provider or the receiver of the service. Since providers of services have very much greater control and power than receivers, it is only too clear who holds all the aces here. In addition, the medical hegemony which still exists in the NHS, despite inroads from general management, ensures that it is doctors' perspectives of quality that are most likely to hold sway. What results then is not quality of health service, but quality of medical service, since for many doctors ill health is still conceptualised through a restricted biomedical model of disease.

If the different professional groups within the health service hold contrary views concerning such fundamental issues as to what health is, it is not surprising that they should conjecture different perceptions on the question of quality. Not only that, but the ultimate consumers of the service – the public – generally have had little opportunity to influence not only the level of quality, but more fundamentally how that quality should be defined. Furthermore, if quality is not an intrinsic attribute but may change according to perspective (both the definitions above implying this), then it is perfectly feasible for quality to yo-yo up and down according to what is currently available.

So it is the consumer of services who defines quality. Although this sounds acceptable its logical extension illustrates the problems associated with such a definition, for it implies that where resources are scarce then, what in a moral argument would not be considered acceptable, becomes just that. In this understanding of quality, if you have been waiting for five years for a hip replacement in an area which has reduced the numbers of this operation to minimal levels, and you manage to make it to the top of the list, you might consider that a quality service had been provided. To attempt to plan services on the basis of these types of definition is thus inherently flawed. To provide services 'of quality' which are genuinely valued by the people who use them requires both a re-examination of what this concept means and a recognition that as things stand quality is defined with reference to existing provision – clearly an undesirable state of affairs.

Planning for quality care

The discussions above, and the similar arguments that were put forward regarding the concept of need, highlight a rather bizarre phenomenon which is becoming more and more familiar to healthcare workers. This is the situation where everybody is being encouraged to use particular words (be they quality, health need, health gain, efficiency, standards and so on – the list is endless), while the meaning of these terms and concepts remains obscure. Somewhere there must be a definition – we just haven't come across it yet. From the above it is apparent that usage of the word quality, and indeed of many of these other words in the NHS, has become distorted. However, planning for quality care cannot proceed without a more insightful exploration of what this concept entails. In his book *Fortress NHS*, Seedhouse (1994) discusses these ideas more fully, and suggests that there are four requisites necessary to make a judgement of quality:

- Standards must exist.
- The purpose of the NHS must be understood.
- In a complex service a range of specific aspects must be evaluated.
- Knowledge and experience of the process being evaluated is required.

Quality does not exist as an absolute – there must be some scale or standard against which it may be compared. Going back to the example of the Belgian chocolates, we are able to describe these as quality chocolates because they may be compared in taste, texture, smell, cocoa content etc. with other chocolate which is not of quality. It is true to say that the audit process does include a comparison of service with a pre-set standard in order to judge quality. Two points need attention here however. Firstly, caution must be exercised in how the standard is set and who has the responsibility for this (see also *Evaluation* in this chapter). Secondly, the fit for purpose definition so often adopted in quality assurance is meaningless here. Applying this to our example, all chocolate, unless it is contaminated with food-poisoning organisms, may be said to be fit for its purpose, i.e. eating, but we do not regard all chocolate as having quality. In other words, some chocolate may be described as of quality and other varieties as below this standard or ordinary.

The second requisite continues a theme which runs throughout this section. It poses the question of whether, without an explicit and collective purpose, rational planning within the NHS is possible. Although it may be possible to determine specific aspects of the quality of particular services, since this must perforce occur in the absence of an overall purpose to the NHS, only a partial judgement of quality is occurring. The NHS is a complex organisation, employing a large and diverse workforce. The range of activities and the different locales in which healthcare may be delivered ensure that quality may be compromised in many different settings and in many different ways. The overall quality of the organisation can only be judged through the assessment of specific elements, but these elements must be representative of the activities that occur. Here quality assurance has followed the same path as much of what occurs under the remit of health services research, for like this latter endeavour quality assurance has tended to focus on activities that are easily measured, and also to focus on outcome rather than process. This is not surprising, since (superficially at least) counting, say, the number of days people stay in hospital or the percentage of 'successful' resections of the prostate is a lot easier, less time-consuming and cheaper than determining what the experience of those people had been or whether in the recipients' terms the hospitalisation for surgery had been a 'quality experience'. This merely re-emphasises the stranglehold that scientific methods in general, and statistics in particular, have on activities within the health service. It raises similar points to those discussed in Chapter 4 concerning the recording of mortality and morbidity rates. This obsession with quantitative measurements has dominated quality assurance and resulted in a restriction of the range of activities being judged.

Finally, it is rather obvious, but needs stating, that quality cannot be judged in the absence of knowledge and experience. This is not to say that doctors are the only ones who should be involved in medical audit, or likewise for nursing. What it does challenge, however, is the notion that quality assurance can be imposed through a structure which ignores the different perspectives that each player in the health service game may have. Certainly the objectives and perceptions of managers, nurses, doctors, carers and patients will differ, but each has a part of the jigsaw to contribute.

Evaluation forms an essential component in the planning cycle, and the assurance of quality is part of this process. A meaningful and comprehensive assessment of quality may be attained only by taking cognisance of the points raised above. If undue emphasis is focused on the quantitative measurement of disease-oriented aspects, then a considerable proportion of what is undertaken in the health service will fail to be captured by the quality assurance process. This is not to dismiss such exercises as worthless – they should form part of any well-conceived plan to evaluate quality. It is obvious that epidemiology will have a considerable role in contributing the methodology for many of the number-counting exercises that are undertaken under this rubric. However, as noted earlier and in Chapter 4, such methods, like any other, have advantages and disadvantages. Appreciating these limitations can only lead to a more rigorous and useful analysis of quality than is currently occurring in the NHS.

More significantly, if the meaning attached to quality remains obscured and the purpose behind the service left unanswered, then, despite much activity and a great deal of money being expended, little will be achieved. As Seedhouse (1994, p. 125) tellingly notes, quality as it is currently perceived 'is associated only with function, and not with moral function. However, once it is understood that working for health is a moral endeavour, quality in healthcare must be associated with a moral function'. While the reasoning underpinning the endeavour remains shrouded in meaningless jargon and illogic, the science of epidemiology may be applied with the utmost rigour but to nil effect.

This chapter on planning and epidemiology has raised a wide variety of issues, some more controversial than others. Given a cursory glance, planning may be regarded as the straightforward application of a series of principles. Although this is undoubtedly the case in a pragmatic sense, some of the material covered in the first section will, it is hoped, serve to stimulate a rather deeper probing into this essentially bureaucratic process. By adopting a polemical approach it is hoped that both sides of the planning process, and by admission the part that epidemiology plays in it, will have been exposed for scrutiny. In some senses it is less easy to appreciate the connection that epidemiology has with planning when compared with its contribution to, say, healthcare assessment. This chapter has certainly proved more difficult to write than those others! It may come as a surprise to some that epidemiology might play a role in such activities as quality assurance or evaluation. It is part of the purpose of this book, however, to uncover those more subtle roles where epidemiology may impinge on the provision of healthcare in general and nursing care in particular.

Snug in its subservient position within the health service hierarchy, nursing has historically been little involved in managing or planning of services. But with the advent of the new nursing, a more proactive and educated rather than trained workforce, nursing is in a position to contribute more to the debates surrounding these issues – issues which in these days of financial stringency and accountability are having a profound effect on the shape of the health service in the 1990s. Unharnessed by a legacy of past endeavours, nursing could campaign for a more democratic and enlightened vision of planning to take forward into the future.

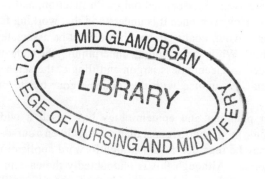

CHAPTER SIX

The application of epidemiology in nursing practice

NURSING QUESTIONS – EPIDEMIOLOGICAL ANSWERS?

For many nurses, epidemiology represents the antithesis of their own discipline. They view it, and some might say rightly so, as a quantitative science heavily influenced and subservient to the tenets of medicine. However, as Chapter 3 of this book outlined, there are some significant areas where epidemiology might make an auspicious contribution to nursing. This chapter will begin by briefly contrasting the approaches that the two disciplines adopt in an attempt to clarify the common ground. The idea of the problematic nature of epidemiology, raised in each of the chapters thus far, will be expanded with particular reference to nursing practice. These ideas will be further developed through a detailed consideration of three areas where nursing and epidemiology might collaborate to their mutual benefit:

- Health technology assessment
- Surveillance and control
- Risk, screening, and prevention

The problematic nature of epidemiology

Orthodox epidemiology firmly embraces the precepts of science and the scientific method. It is thus driven by positivism, which is a philosophy based on the recognition of positive facts and observable phenomena. Positivism seeks to make specific claims about reality, claims which are objective, empirical and generalisable. Taking a positivist approach, hypotheses are generated, valid data are collected through unbiased observation, and the disinterested scientist makes inferences based on these data (see Chapter 2). In this way, carefully controlled 'senses' are used to observe and measure 'facts', which become the basis for refuting and testing hypotheses. Science is presented therefore as a value-free enterprise: objective and neutral, with the path to truth unobstructed by emotion or bias. Political and ideological perspectives do not (it is claimed) enter this equation. For positivist epidemiology therefore, 'human disease is an observable, biological fact and is subject to cause and effect regularities which involve other observable phenomena' (Jones and Moon, 1987, p. 311).

An alternative perspective to positivism is provided by *naturalism/interpretism*, which opines that social worlds cannot be broken down into a series of objects that can be validly and accurately measured. Instead, things are studied 'as they are', since, it is contended, different things have different meanings for different people. In other words, people make the worlds they live in and there is no objective reality. Meaning does not have a fixed entity, but may change depending on context (time and place). The universal cause and effect relationships posited by traditional epidemiology are difficult to reconcile with this other way of viewing the world, or this other paradigm. If there are multiple perspectives on a problem, and these may change with time and place, then is it possible to set up generalisable laws which purport to predict cause and effect relationships?

During the last thirty years the impetus for a third view of social theory has grown. Developed through Hegelian philosophy, *critical theory* centres on the belief that knowledge evolves through the human ability to act rationally to achieve a greater knowledge and emancipation of the self. One of its principle tenets concerns how reflection on the conditions and reasons that limit actions leads to emancipation and transformation. Moving beyond the notions of objectivity and measurability encompassed in positivism, and the naturalistic school of thought, where understanding is based on an interpretation of social interactions, critical perspectives are founded in the neo-Marxist thinking of the Frankfurt school (Habermas, 1971). Causality is thus redefined not through empiricism and positivism, but on realism and materialism.

A new theory enmeshed within the idea of the social production of illness and health thus emerges. Its philosophy – realism – seeks explanations in terms of the underpinning structures and mechanisms which may either inhibit or promote certain changes. For example, it is not enough to know that a relationship exists between low social class and smoking; a realist epidemiology seeks to understand the social structures that explain why this is. Critical epidemiology argues that the major causes of health inequality are to be found not in the body, nor in individual personal behaviour, but in the ways by which society is organised (Jones and Moon, 1987). As these authors note

(1987, p. 316), '...an epidemiology that concentrates on individual level explanations and does not consider the basic structure of society as in any way problematic mystifies the social origins of disease and legitimates the status quo'.

A new approach

A theory that acknowledges the social production of sickness and indeed health will require a redefinition of causality. Unlike positivism, which contends that causation is linked with regularity, realism accepts that certain changing conditions dictate that single events are no less 'caused' than multiple events. What causes something to happen has nothing to do with the number of times it has happened or been observed to happen, and hence whether it constitutes regularity (Sayer, 1984, p. 162). Similarly, the positivist rule that cause precedes effect and that there is a regularity among events is challenged by Marxist thinking, which proposes that conjunction is not constant but organic. Nature and society are open systems where reciprocal effects predominate (Turshen, 1989). The logical end-point of an espousal of open systems is the rejection of the deductive and inductive theories of science and an affirmation that social studies can only ever be explanatory and not predictive. In addition, open systems acknowledge the existence of structures and emergent powers that may limit individual action. In contrast, positivism has presumed that by understanding the individual, society may be understood.

A critical epidemiology must also re-examine the ideas surrounding disease classifications, which are currently based upon technical biological criteria (Chapter 2). The social construction of sickness suggests that rather than being fixed and universal, 'diseases' are shaped by society, and particularly by those in power in society. Through this classification diseases could be defined by their common social origins. Draper *et al.* (1977) provide just such a classification, where the aetiology and risk factors for disease fall into such categories as 'How we share'. Here risk factors, such as inadequate housing and lack of basic amenities, which persist despite increasing levels of productivity, result in respiratory and gastro-intestinal diseases. The reclassification of diseases based on social origins is discussed also by Cameron and Jones (1985). They describe how people use legal and illegal drugs to treat a variety of dis-eases such as boredom, anxiety and incompetence. As Jones and Moon (1987, p. 322) note, 'They [diseases] must be examined as contingent and historically specific struggles over who, and for what purpose, provides the definition and makes the diagnosis'.

Another fundamental question concerns what the unit of analysis should be, for epidemiology, like nursing, takes the individual as its basic unit, but then attempts to generalise to a larger population. This reductionist approach denies the social context in which such individuals are situated and attempts to explain the collective merely as the sum of all its individual components. For example, the risk of getting a pressure sore during hospitalisation is not only to be explained in terms of individual nutritional status and skin condition, but is also dependent on the length of time patients spend lying on hard surfaces in Accident and Emergency departments while awaiting admission. This in its turn is related to political and economic policies concerning the provision of healthcare and, specifically, of hospital beds.

Similarly the taxonomic collectives with which epidemiologists traditionally work may not possess any functional reality. In other words, the groups that epidemiologists use or construct in the course of their work may not be an accurate reflection of the true state of affairs. An example of this is the use of occupation to denote social class. This system of social stratification has frequently been challenged, and other classifications based on, for example, income or education, may be more appropriate. Similarly the use of chronological age groups such as the 'young old' (under 75 years of age) and the 'old old' (over 75 years of age) creates misleading stereotypes – the former hale and hearty and the latter sick and decrepit – and often bears little resemblance to the disparate and variable experiences of different individuals of these ages.

Another hallmark of mainstream epidemiology is its almost total reliance on quantitative methodologies, which are often characterised by large sample sizes. Although many subjects may be studied, the data collected will often be relatively superficial and highly categorised. Some examples might be social class, sex, number of children, years of secondary education and such like. This is in direct contrast to qualitative approaches, which may study only a few cases, but study them in depth. These latter designs are dismissed by positivists as anecdotal evidence.

These differences are not merely methodological: they also usually reflect a fundamental difference in epistemologies between the two research traditions. Empirical science believes that the social world is amenable to measurement and experimentation, and as such it usually utilises quantitative methodologies. In order both to measure phenomena quantitatively and to predict through empirical regularities, social processes are treated as things (reification). These things must remain static and not change their nature over time. This assumes that social systems are closed and the existing relationships captured at one moment in time represent the natural state of affairs. From this particular world view, rigorous research is achieved through standardised interpretation and the prior categorisation of the elements of the phenomenon under investigation. Objective collection of data by the researcher, who remains 'immune' from the process being undertaking, is also required.

In contrast, qualitative designs are usually espoused by those whose paradigm encompasses the ideas that social systems are open and ever-changing. In order to gain an understanding of any particular situation it is therefore necessary to obtain much deeper and richer information. The prior setting of categories by the researcher is anathema to this approach: categories will 'emerge' from the data as it is collected.

In addition, many qualitative approaches contend that the researcher will always have an effect on data collection. Moral, ethical and political influences centring on how the project was funded, who and how the original questions were posed, the cultural environment of the work – these will all influence how researchers will conduct and interpret their work.

From this standpoint research cannot be shaken free from the context and the values of the environment in which it is conceived and conducted. A further description and exploration of these ideas may be found in Latour and Woolgar's account (1979) of the social production of biological facts, and Ratcliffe and Gonzalez del Valle's critique (1988) of rigour in health-related research. Qualitative designs are epitomised by ethnography, which attempts to understand social situations through the eye of the beholder. The researcher, far from being objective, enters into an interactive and non-hierarchical relationship with respondents with the latter rather than the former driving the research agenda. Proponents of qualitative methods insist that it is only by such interactive and intensive methods that some of the reality of dynamic human systems can be described.

It is clear from the foregoing that particular paradigms will determine both how the world is viewed and the 'best' methods through which research investigations should proceed. Orthodox epidemiology has adopted one particular paradigm and therefore for many social scientists suffers from a number of problems. Its unquestioning acceptance of biomedicine and its underlying philosophies of positivism and reductionism create difficulties when investigations move outside the control of the laboratory and into the social world. These problems are both epistemological and methodological. The espousal of one system of disease classification, and indeed the reification of diseases into 'things', pushes epidemiology into the pursuit of biological explanations and, in particular, individual explanations for sickness.

In the face of undeniable evidence that diseases are not merely biological phenomena, but exist in a certain time and place according to prevailing social conditions, the adoption of a biomedical model precludes all but a rudimentary analysis of the other factors which might impinge upon sickness. By reifying and compartmentalising social processes into neat categories these attributes are portrayed as immutable and thereby beyond changing. The categories provide the framework for describing the unequal distribution of sickness, but by ignoring critical perspectives, mainstream epidemiology then seeks answers to these differences at the level of the individual, rather than the level of society. These epistemological concerns are perpetuated through the quantitative methods used to seek explanations. By their very construction these methods preclude any meaningful analysis of social processes, separating as they do experience from phenomena. Instead, they provide a 'description of momentary regularities literally plucked out of a much larger explanatory structure... a snapshot of the interrelationships' (Pawson, 1978, p.624).

The questions facing epidemiology now are whether a more critical perspective and/or an interpretative stance could enhance the field of enquiry beyond its biomedical origins. This has important implications for nursing, since many within the profession already contend that the social world of sickness and health cannot be investigated solely through the paradigms and methods of empirical science (Duffy, 1985; Melia, 1982). An epidemiology which began to explore questions of sickness and health from these different epistemological and methodological perspectives would have much more in common with many of the prevailing ideologies in nursing. In addition, this convergence of thinking might enable nursing to reciprocate and offer in its turn some grist for the epidemiological mill. Nursing, after all, does not hold the same philosophies and aims of medicine. Should not a universal epidemiology be exploring questions of sickness and health through a framework that nursing holds important too?

Epidemiology and nursing: is there a common ground?

Since many nurses will not be given the opportunity to study epidemiology during training, their experience of this discipline may either be non-existent or be mediated through their professional contact with medical colleagues. This may promote one particular view of epidemiology, strongly linked to biomedicine, the disease model of health, and quantitative methods. Many nurses therefore, and indeed many epidemiologists, may either reject or remain in ignorance of the critical and interpretive perspectives discussed in the preceding section – questions probing the validity of classification systems, the unit of analysis and the strategy for obtaining information are not raised in a biomedical hegemony embedded in positivism (see Chapters 1 and 2). In addition, although, unlike biomedicine, orthodox epidemiology does recognise factors external to the body which may cause sickness, the operationalisation of these concepts is narrow and primitive.

Despite the inclusion of 'social factors' in epidemiological studies, there is rarely any sociological input into their conceptualisation (Spruit and Kromhoult, 1987). The complex, multifaceted and ever-changing phenomenon which is society is reduced to immutable categories (such as social class, racial origin, level of income) that are fixed in time and space. Furthermore, the analysis usually stops at the individual, thus excluding prior societal and structural variables. A critical perspective that acknowledges these aspects is therefore lacking. Nursing has traditionally given scant attention to the socio-economic and political perspectives of its position and work. It comes as no surprise therefore that the arguments for a critical perspective outlined above have received little or no attention.

It has been mentioned earlier that nursing could hold a privileged position with regard to the possibilities of taking a fresh view of epidemiology. To date, any successful adoption or incorporation of epidemiology within nursing has been constrained by two factors. Firstly, the mediation of information concerning the discipline through the channels of biomedicine has led many nurses to discard outright epidemiological methods and models. Secondly, for nursing it is the individual who remains central to the field of focus. This latter philosophy tends to subvert any theories that point to the importance of factors beyond the individual, such as political or economic conditions, in the genesis of sickness. A critical epidemiology, which might at face value mesh more smoothly with the ideologies of nursing, may struggle in this environment.

However, as a young discipline nursing holds some advantages. Although many commentators have bemoaned the continuing and often acrimonious debate within nursing concerning its rightful subject matter and the research designs that it should adopt, critical and open discussions foster new and innovative approaches. Furthermore, being in a unique position *vis-á-vis* those other central players – the doctors – nursing may hold the conceptual keys to enriching and widening the epidemiological tradition in healthcare, for nursing has largely unharnessed itself from the biomedical model of disease, and yet is still intricately entwined with medicine and its practitioners.

Despite shedding its handmaiden image, the reality of nursing certainly encompasses a significant element of administering the 'doctor's orders', be these for a drug, a specific treatment or a course of action, such as discharge from hospital, or bed rest.

Nevertheless nursing has its own particular objectives and frameworks through which it acts. Based on the principle of individualised care and the notion of holism, nursing moves beyond biomedicine into more complex areas where the definition of causality lies well beyond reductionist views of biological abnormalities within the body. Although the focus and application of epidemiology and nursing may be different, the former's espousal of a holistic framework for studying the spectrum of health and illness aligns the two enterprises. Epidemiology focuses on how the well-being of humans is affected by their physical, social and cultural environments, and in this sense it is much closer to nursing then to medicine. It has a wide concern, encompassing the multifactorial webs of causation for both chronic and acute afflictions. Rather than sweeping epidemiology into the untouchable box that is biomedicine, nursing needs to avail itself of epidemiological perspectives and methodologies lest a valuable opportunity to move in new and essential directions is lost. Nursing and nurses are in a pivotal position to both enrich their own discipline and to contribute to a wider and more realistic interpretation of epidemiology.

APPLYING EPIDEMIOLOGY IN NURSING PRACTICE

Thus far this chapter has attempted to situate the relative positions of epidemiology and nursing. Through an exploration of the limitations of epidemiology as it is currently practised some avenues through which these difficulties might be resolved have been described. The idea of a closer relationship between nursing and epidemiology fostered through a more open recognition of the problems that face a truly social epidemiology was proposed. Each discipline, nursing and epidemiology, has its own paradigms, fields of knowledge, requirements and objectives, and yet crucially they retain a similar goal focused on the well-being of humans and how this may be affected by physical, social and cultural factors.

This section will describe three areas where a union between these two disciplines might enhance either enterprise or both. It should be stressed here (and this sentiment is echoed throughout this book) that epidemiology has a much broader relevance to nursing than the exploration that these three topics allow. These particular topics were chosen for two reasons: firstly, their particular historical and ongoing relevance for each discipline, and secondly their current importance to the philosophical and organisational changes that the NHS has undergone in the last decade. It is clear, however, that nurses working within all spheres of the profession would benefit both from a greater recognition of the benefits that an 'epidemiological eye' may bring and also from an enhanced appreciation of where epidemiology (at least in its traditional model) may provide either an incomplete or distorted understanding of the aetiology and control of sickness.

Health technology assessment (HTA)

In considering the contribution that epidemiology might make to nursing, Chapter 3 examined some of the issues involved in clinical decision-making. Although touching upon decision analysis in its purest sense, it was suggested that a more general interest in the ways in which nurses collect and use information to govern their decisions in clinical practice was more appropriate to this book. In particular, the recent governmental concern with maximising the efficiency and effectiveness of healthcare through the auspices of the restructured NHS was emphasised. Here efficiency is defined as the 'ability of a healthcare intervention to produce the desired outcome in a defined population under ideal conditions. Effectiveness is the extent to which that outcome is achieved under the usual conditions of care in "real life"...' (Hopkins, 1993, p. 117).

Health technologies have been defined in a recent report (Department of Health, 1992b, p. 8) to include 'all the methods used by healthcare professionals to promote health, to prevent and treat disease, and to improve rehabilitation and long term care'. Both hardware, such as equipment, and software, such as diagnostic policies and educational strategies were included in the definition. It was proposed that rigorous assessment of technologies was crucial in establishing 'their effectiveness and safety, their cost effectiveness and their social and organisational impacts' (Department of Health, 1992b, p. 8). The criticisms of the NHS reforms and the concerns that such evaluations will centre on economic issues notwithstanding, it is clear that health technology assessment (HTA) will play a major role in nursing research and development for the foreseeable future. Indeed the evaluation of the effectiveness of clinical procedures, practices and interventions is seen as the fundamental research task for nursing in the *Report of the Taskforce on the Strategy for Research in Nursing, Midwifery and Health Visiting* (Department of Health, 1993a).

This same report emphasised the fiscal and staffing implications of nursing in the health service. Collectively, nurses account for one third of health authorities' expenditures, and they represent the largest professional body within the NHS. As the report notes, 'Purchasers, providers and managers... need reliable data on the nursing contribution to health gain and patient care if such a large workforce is to be used to maximum benefit' (Department of Health, 1993a, p. 8). Within this framework, research into the efficiency and effectiveness of clinical interventions is essential. The report also makes it clear that some considerable effort will be required to establish outcome measures. The issues that nursing must address in HTA, and the opportunities for epidemiology to participate in the framing and answering of the questions that may arise, fall into three areas:

- the identification of nursing practices that require evaluation
- the selection of research designs appropriate to evaluating those interventions
- the development of outcome measures

The identification of nursing practices that require evaluation.

It does not require very much thought to devise a long list of nursing practices that could usefully be subject to a rigorous appraisal. In addition, it is clear that there are different categories of clinical procedures, practices and interventions which may require different research approaches to their evaluation. These activities range from undertaking easily recognisable treatments, such as bladder washouts, mouth care or wound cleansing, and the provision of equipment such as urethral catheters, walking aids, pressure-relieving mattresses and the like, to less easily defined practices, such as providing information, spiritual and moral support, and health promotion advice. Alongside these practice issues are other more global concerns, such as the strategies through which nursing care should be delivered.

However, a finite budget demands that decisions must be made as to which areas of health technology should take priority in any assessment programme. Again, within these areas choices are required to identify those practices or interventions that would most benefit from evaluation. Generally, priorities should be approached through a framework that makes clinical and social needs and value for money the moving forces (Department of Health, 1992b). Three dimensions must be addressed: the social and political importance of the problem, the possibility of improving patient outcomes and the potential for achieving any answers through research. Since in the UK the major funder of nursing research is the Department of Health, it is likely that the setting of priorities will closely follow governmental policies and concerns. These have been outlined in *The Health of the Nation*

(Department of Health, 1992a) and *Research for Health* (Department of Health, 1993h) which summarise the direction of the Department of Health's research and development strategy, including the contribution of health technology assessment. Refreshingly, it is clear that at least in part these strategies are now taking into account the differing perspectives that different professionals – managers, doctors, nurses, policy-makers – and the lay public may have on what constitutes a priority area.

However, the need for nursing to be proactive is crucial. The HTA advisory group was notable for its lack of nursing membership. The report produced by this group emphasises that 'for each major **disease or speciality** it will be necessary to list the existing and anticipated preventative and therapeutic approaches and the skills they require; to estimate the efficacy and hazards of these health technologies; and to judge whether they are worth their cost' (Department of Health, 1992b, p. 9). This approach is advocated to produce a 'shopping list' of research questions worthy of priority funding. Although there is nothing intrinsically wrong with this strategy, nursing must take warning of two caveats. Firstly, it is essential that an informed nursing perspective is included in priority-setting in HTA. Secondly, nursing must recognise that the framework through which the NHS health strategy and thus its research priorities is formulated is still heavily embedded in a biomedical agenda. For example, four of the five *Health of the Nation* key target areas are constructed through a biomedical disease classification (coronary heart disease and stroke; cancers; mental illness; HIV/AIDS). To pick up the example from above, which called on Draper *et al.*'s (1977) new classification of sickness, there is no target concerned with 'How we share' and its effect on the health of UK citizens.

Similarly, the emphasis on discrete, bounded patient groups, such as the 'elderly', or 'mother and child' perpetuates the conventional epidemiological tendencies to group what may be highly disparate people together according to convenient, but perhaps meaningless, labels. Put another way, it may be rather difficult to frame and conduct research studies that pursue a genuine social epidemiological remit when biomedicine remains as the hegemonic socio-political research culture. These are some of the more covert and global issues that nurses and other healthcare professionals need to be aware of in the area of health technology assessment. However, to give hope to the faint-hearted, this particular section will end with some examples of where HTAs have already been successfully pursued in nursing.

Randomised controlled trials (RCTs) remain the benchmark for HTA. Although widely used in medicine, such designs have been less extensively used in nursing. However, a number of well-documented studies evaluating the merit of certain interventions or systems of delivering care instigated by midwives are witnessed by the work of the National Perinatal Epidemiology Unit (NPEU) at Oxford. Perhaps the best known of these is the randomised controlled trial conducted by Sleep *et al.* (1984) comparing two perineal management policies during spontaneous vaginal delivery. The policies, which were both intended to minimise trauma, involved either the restrictive or liberal use of episiotomy. One thousand women were recruited and randomly allocated to one of the two groups. Significantly more of the woman allocated to the liberal rather than the restrictive policy required suturing for perineal tears post delivery. This study has had a considerable impact upon midwifery care.

Other RCTs undertaken by midwives in conjunction with NPEU include a comparison of different materials for suture of the perineum (Mahomed *et al.*, 1989); the effect of an obstetric birth chair on delivery (Crowley *et al.*, 1991); and a comparison of breast shells and Hoffman's exercises for inverted and non-protractile nipples (Alexander *et al.*, 1992). These studies indicate that midwifery care is just as amenable to evaluation through randomised controlled trials as is medical care.

Wilson-Barnett and Batehup (1988) provide further examples of where experimental research has produced the evidence on which guidelines for practice may be based. However, such experimental designs are not widely utilised by nurse researchers. An analysis of articles published in the *Journal of Advanced Nursing* noted that the number of research studies that used an experimental or quasi-experimental approach fell from 21% in 1981 to 15% in 1991 (Mulhall, 1994). As noted in Chapter 1, where nurses have used epidemiological approaches to research cohort designs have found greater favour than RCTs. Observational approaches such as cohort studies may be used for HTA, but only, it is suggested, where the effect of the technology is large, or where RCTs are not feasible (Department of Health, 1992b). This question of appropriate methodologies will be discussed further in the next section.

What is worth noting here is that, where RCTs have been used for HTA within nursing, the research has often essentially assumed a biomedical or quasi-biomedical framework. Outcomes have generally been operationalised in terms of concrete biological or physiological phenomena, for example the need for suturing after delivery. The very nature of trials, couched as they are in positivism, demands that such measurable and objective outcomes are available. The emphasis in medicine on diagnosis and treatment lends itself more readily to an

HTA that embraces such approaches. The use of RCTs for HTA within nursing may be more problematic and this is an issue which will be explored below and in the section which considers outcomes.

There are, however, many instances where the questions being posed within nursing can be usefully operationalised and measured using objective scientific methodologies. Many of the technical procedures undertaken and the equipment used during the provision of nursing care could usefully be examined for their efficiency and effectiveness using RCTs. Some of the questions that are continually being posed by practitioners are 'Which bladder washout should I use when a urethral catheter is blocked? Is this cheaper disinfectant equally as effective as the one in current use? Will a new pressure-relieving mattress prevent pressure sores? Should the insertion sites of intravenous cannulae be covered by sterile dressings? Questions such as these can be effectively tackled through the framework of experimental research, i.e. through clinical trials. These are areas where technical outcomes are normally the most relevant and appropriate – a patient with a blocked catheter has one pressing objective, which is to be relieved of the physical pain of urinary retention. Similarly, patients undergoing intravenous therapy will be rather keen to avoid the potential life-threatening side-effect of infection. In this instance, therefore, a biological outcome measure is highly significant to the patient, and any investigation of the effectiveness of various dressings would rightly include infection as a primary outcome measure.

Research designs and HTA

Within the framework of the natural sciences any reliable assessment of the effects of a particular healthcare practice must attempt to minimise systematic errors (or bias) and random errors (or chance). Conventional methods for evaluating the effects of healthcare may be divided into two categories: observational designs, such as cohort studies and case-controlled designs, which use statistical techniques to control for selection bias (see Chapter 1), and experimental approaches, such as RCTs, which allocate patients at random to two groups with the aim of eliminating bias at this stage (see Chapter 1 for an explanation of these terms and designs). It has been suggested that while the moderate biases to which observational studies are prone would be acceptable if the effect of a technology is large, 'strict randomisation, analysis and interpretation, without bias, is usually necessary' to detect more moderate effects (Department of Health, 1992b, p. 14).

However, as noted above, the use of RCTs within nursing research has been quite limited, and the question of why this should be requires some attention. An easy reply, which probably contains some elements of the truth, is that nursing has no firmly embedded tradition of using experimental designs, and nurses receive little pre- or post-registration training in the techniques necessary to conduct such studies. Alternatively, the practical and conceptual framework through which nursing acts may preclude such approaches or limit their usefulness. Does this mean that health technology assessment in nursing should be abandoned because the benchmark design for medicine, i.e. the RCT, is not appropriate in many cases, and in addition few nurses are able to undertake or appreciate these designs? Or could alternative designs more congruent with the philosophy and aims of nursing provide a suitable alternative? The answer probably lies between the two. Certainly there is no reason why, with better opportunities for training and a wider participation in multidisciplinary research teams, nurses should not capitalise on experimental epidemiological methods and use them when appropriate for HTA in nursing. But as Andrews (1991, p. 5) notes, '...the randomised controlled trial is a tool to be used, not a god to be worshipped'.

This same author describes the limitations of RCTs in one particular branch of medicine – rehabilitation. The comments that he makes are pertinent, for they also generally apply to many of the interventions or 'therapies' that nursing utilises. Andrews notes a number of difficulties related to 'the treatment'. Some aspects of rehabilitation, such as ultrasound or transcutaneous electrical nerve stimulation, offer the possibility for defining discrete treatments, but many other aspects of care cannot be so easily packaged. Similarly, nursing involves some procedures that are well-defined and bounded, but many others where a tight definition of what is occurring would be difficult. In addition, attempts to standardise the treatment dosage, while easy enough for drugs, is much more difficult when comparing processes such as time spent with the physiotherapist, how bed-bound patients are turned to prevent pressure sores, the giving of information prior to surgery and so on.

The question of patient and investigator blinding is also generally problematic when the nature of the technology, either soft, or hard, is obvious. For example, Bainton *et al.* (1982) compared two types of pads for urinary incontinence. However, the type of pad being used would have been obvious both to the client and the investigator, thus introducing a source of bias to the study.

Finally, nursing, by adopting a philosophy of holism, is very aware of the continual interactions that occur between the different systems surrounding and composing the body of those in their care. The balance of physiological and structural systems, the interactions and fusion of mind and body, and the effect of the environment and sociocultural milieu of the caring encounter may all be interacting to a greater or lesser extent at any specific moment. Attempts to reduce such multisytems down to discrete observable units so that groups with comparable characteristics may be compared seem almost impossible. In other words, the very uniqueness in time and space of any particular intervention, and thus its outcome, would indicate the presence of multiple complicating variables, which in a conventional RCT would need balancing out.

There are partial solutions to some of these limitations to the use of RCTs for HTA in nursing. The question of non-blinding, which often occurs in healthcare research, can be tackled to some extent by taking extreme precautions when evaluating outcomes, and, where subjects are likely to favour one treatment over another, to employ a crossover design. Using this latter strategy subjects may at least be reassured that they will receive the test treatment either straight away or after a short delay.

The definition of treatments which are multifaceted cannot necessarily be resolved, but by taking a 'pragmatic' approach to trial design difficulties may be minimised (Swartz *et al.*, 1980). In pragmatic trials, comparisons are made under conditions that might normally prevail in practice, and thus some deviation from the 'treatment' is allowable as long as the analysis is based on 'intention to treat', i.e. for the analysis subjects remain in the group to which they are allocated regardless of which 'treatment' they actually receive. In this way random allocation is retained. Bond *et al.* (1989a,b) describe the use of a pragmatic approach to a randomised controlled trial of institutionalised care for the elderly, where capturing the process of care (the staff/patient interactions, the unwritten rules and regulations, the sociocultural environment) and determining how it affected outcome was far from straightforward.

In many drug trials, while elaborate precautions are in place to ensure strict randomisation, physical comparability of the drug and placebo, and blinded outcome evaluations, scant attention has been paid to other sociocultural factors which may affect a subject's response. If factors beyond the pharmacological properties of a drug and its mere ingestion (as drug or placebo), such as when, how and by whom it is given, may influence outcome, then the 'context' in which drugs are provided requires careful standardisation.

Conventional trials focus their spotlight on outcomes. Trials that involve the evaluation of healthcare in general and nursing care specifically need to take more cognisance of the process of care. Greater heed of Donabedian's comment (1980, p. 81) that, 'the most direct route to an assessment of the quality of care is an examination of that care' might produce more meaningful results. In this context, Newell (1992), describing both the study by Bond *et al.* (1989a,b) and another trial investigating the optimum length of hospital stay following minor surgery (Russell *et al.* 1977) emphasises the requirement for a multidisciplinary team (in this case people with training in statistics, medicine, nursing, sociology, economics, computing and anthropology). Such teams are able to demonstrate methodological flexibility and provide a qualitative aspect to an essentially quantitative design. This type of approach would seem suitable for tackling the type of HTA that nursing may need to undertake. As Newell notes (1992, p. 56), the 'pragmatic approach in the trial can lead to the conclusion "provide this package of services and produce better survival or personal well-being", the qualitative method attempts to unwrap the package "unravelling the web to determine which aspects of the package are important"'.

A further illustration of the benefits of multidisciplinary research and the relevance of qualitative methods is provided by an evaluation undertaken by Daly *et al.* (1992) of one particular medical technology – echocardiography. This study is referred to in greater detail in the following section.

The development of outcome measures

Classic accounts of randomised trials discuss the concept of the primary response variable – the outcome that is measured during the trial. The primary response variable should define and answer the primary question posed by the trial. For many of the health technologies that medicine uses, outcome measures have often been defined in terms of morbidity or mortality. This accords well both with medical practitioners' concern with cure, and with medicine's adoption of positivistic science as its ostensible foundation. Although such outcomes would appear clear-cut, there are however, certain methodological challenges in defining such events and ensuring that they are rigorously measured (Haynes, 1988).

In contrast with medicine, nursing has a care orientation that is not as heavily focused on physical or psychological improvements. Caring is concerned with providing the support necessary to allow improvement, maintain the *status quo* or ensure a pain-free and dignified death. Despite these differences in philosophical basis and *modus operandi*, much nursing technology could profitably adopt outcomes similar to those traditionally utilised by medicine.

There are, however, limitations to such rigid outcomes. Take a seemingly straightforward example, the trial of a new bladder washout purported to prevent urinary encrustations on catheters. It might be suggested that the primary outcome variable should be the dry weight of inorganic material found on the catheters of those who were or were not treated with this new product. However, even this simple example illustrates some of the difficulties that may be encountered in attempting to define and measure meaningful outcome measures. A meaningful evaluation of this new technology would need to determine not just the dry weight of the encrustation, but also its effect on the function of the catheter. Perhaps the distribution of the deposits is more important, or their chemical composition, or some other unknown physiological variable associated with the patient's urine. In addition, the reliability of this measure might be compromised, since the physical removal of the catheter may dislodge encrustations, and the factors affecting this, such as operator error and patient compliance, may be uncontrollable. It is clear, therefore, that in both medicine and nursing carefully defined and rigidly bounded biological outcomes may be appropriate, but often this will not absolve investigators from a range of methodological challenges.

The evaluation of healthcare technologies is, however, a wider enterprise. Where the design of an evaluation is simple, and the factors involved relatively specific, such as in studies of a single bodily organ, a drug or a biochemical response, then RCTs with traditional outcome measures may suffice. However, increasingly even these types of study are being questioned in terms of the validity and appropriateness of their outcome measures. At the heart of this disquiet lie two fundamental questions:

- Who should decide what is appropriate in terms of outcome?
- Is it outcome or process which is important?

HTA has, until recently, been restricted to a largely medical domain, and continues to be overlaid by a medical hegemony. The contingencies of the internal market and the development of a research strategy for the NHS have led the drive towards a greater emphasis upon the efficiency and effectiveness of services. This has not only opened up the question of how all types of health technology might be evaluated, but has broadened the debate to include other practitioners, such as nurses, physiotherapists and allied professions. However, for nursing to get even a peep around the door two things will be necessary. Firstly, nurses must be able to confidently critique and appreciate the research designs and outcome measures that have been used to date. Secondly, the profession must consider the two questions raised above, and ensure that a nursing dimension is included in any debate.

A thorough understanding and appreciation of the limitations and possibilities offered by epidemiology will be crucial to achieving these two objectives. It is not sufficient to reject epidemiological methods of HTA simply on the grounds that they are biomedically oriented. More imaginative strategies and suggestions congruent with nursing's agenda and philosophies need to be interposed into the arguments. From this viewpoint, the reorganisation of the NHS and its research strategy provides nursing with the opportunity to be included in the debate, but it must be an 'informed' opportunity and an 'informed' input. In other words, the structure and organisation of HTA developments must include nurses and nursing, and the profession in its turn must be capable of informing and broadening the debate.

The question of who decides what is appropriate in terms of outcome measures echoes much of the discussion in Chapter 2 concerning different actors' perceptions of health and sickness. As Hopkins (1993, p. 117) cautions, 'outcomes are complex and multidimensional'. However, as a result of the increasing awareness and necessity for clinical audit much has been written about outcome measures in terms of who provides the input. Thus there may be medical outcomes, nursing outcomes, patient outcomes and even organisational outcomes.

This in a sense muddies the issue, since audit is concerned with the quality of care, professional performance and value for money. While these may be important considerations in HTA, the efficiency and effectiveness of individual contributions to an overall health technology should not be the only criteria through which evaluation takes place. Doctors, nurses, physiotherapists, dietitians, porters, cleaners, managers, receptionists, relatives and friends: all may impinge upon an individual's experience of healthcare and its associated technologies at any particular moment in time.

Within the dynamics of social life, is it possible, or even desirable, to pinpoint particular outcomes and then try to relate them back to a specific input provided by a specific profession? This is not to say that important medical outcomes, such as mortality or physical and physiological functioning and the cataloguing of related side-effects, should be abandoned. These are important outcomes, but they are not the only outcomes. A more reasonable course would be a careful integration of outcome measures that (a) answer medicine's questions and thus provide for a more generalisable body of medical knowledge, and (b) address individual patients' and society's concerns in order that technologies are evaluated in terms more appropriate to consumers' priorities.

The emphasis on consumer choice and satisfaction instigated by the *Patient's Charter* (Department of Health, 1991c) has coerced health professionals into considering these latter viewpoints. A UK Clearing House for Information on the Assessment of Health Outcomes has been established, and outcomes research increasingly guides practice. This research needs to combine information about the likely outcome of different treatments with what matters to the individual recipients of those procedures (Delamothe, 1994). Such data may also be used in planning, but great care must be exercised to ensure that user views are both valid and representative (see Chapter 5). In this respect it is interesting to note that the report from the advisory group on HTA (Department of Health, 1992b), convened by the Department of Health's Director of Research and Development, emphasises the importance of outcomes which 'patients themselves would find interesting[!] and important' (author's exclamation). However, the majority of this document heavily emphasises medical technologies, is peppered with examples from medicine, and frequently reverts to a biomedical agenda. For example, to illustrate how observational studies may contribute to HTA, a discussion of the surgical options available for benign hypertrophy of the prostate is pursued. Yet the studies cited to illustrate the case revert to mortality as the outcome measure.

It is obvious that much needs to be done both to ensure that more than lip service is paid to these new ideas, and also to develop strategies through which consumer perspectives may be canvassed and subsequently incorporated into any evaluation.

In general, much healthcare research is unlikely to avail the investigator with clear-cut end-points that may be used as outcome measures. Similarly, specific nursing interventions usually have very diffuse or hard-to-define outcomes which may only be realised in the long term. Outcome measures that can be validly and reliably measured by scientific methods are not particularly obvious in these settings. In reality, it is difficult to see how any health technology, however small and discrete it might be, can be usefully evaluated once it is torn from the context in which it occurs.

This raises the second question posed above. Is it outcome, or process which is more important? Alongside this runs a parallel debate concerned with identifying the most appropriate methodologies through which HTA should proceed. Conventional epidemiology supports the case for outcomes, and moreover would favour RCTs above other methodologies wherever they are feasible. This idolatry of method and epistemology is clearly indicated by a quote from the report cited above. 'A scientific evaluation depends on having one or more quantifiable outcome measures'. (Department of Health, 1992b, p. 10). This commits HTA to the tenets of science and to quantitative techniques.

However, other options are available and they may be particularly suited to teasing out what is going on during the process of care. Newell (1992) describes how in the study of nursing homes both final outcomes, such as survival and quality of life, and intermediate outcomes, such as type and level of activity of the residents, were considered important. This research utilised not only a randomised controlled trial but six other linked studies. One of these in particular used an ethnographic approach to provide analytical descriptions and comparisons of the modes of care under the two regimes.

This raises another point regarding methodology. Biomedicine has become more flexible in its range of outcome measures, now perceiving such measures as quality of life, the experience of patients and their carers, and personal well-being, as important. However, this flexibility has not extended to how these new outcomes should be measured. It should come as no surprise that, despite the difficulties in ascertaining the validity and reliability of many psycho-social rating scales, it is these instruments that are being used. The nursing home study above provides a notable exception of where positivistic methods have run alongside more interpretative qualitative approaches, such as ethnography. With its more eclectic approach to research, nursing has for many years been adopting and refining such qualitative methods, and it is significant that it was a nurse who conducted the ethnography in the nursing home study. Here then is another opportunity for nursing to provide of its unique experience to enrich the traditional methodologies of HTA.

Pope and Mays (1994, p. 153) in their imaginary dialogue between a sociologist and the director of a health services research unit provide a lively account of the varying perspectives that different disciplines may take to this argument of process versus outcome. As they note, health services research seems to have overlooked 'the part of the action where all the fine words in the policy documents get implemented'. Their argument in a nutshell is what is the point in knowing about outcome if you don't know how you got there? This is amply illustrated by some research which sought to evaluate a particular diagnostic test – echocardiography (Daly *et al.*, 1992). Initially a quasi-experimental design was used to determine the effect of an electrocardiographic test on the care of patients in routine clinical practice (McDonald *et al.*, 1988). This investigation indicated that the test had only a moderate impact on clinical decisions, and that despite receiving a normal test result patients returned repeatedly for further reassurance. Thus this quantitative study revealed a number of difficulties which could not be answered satisfactorily within its design.

At this point the researchers considered conducting a randomised trial with an outcome measure of 'reassurance'. Although there were ethical and practical problems for this approach, it was not adopted for another reason. The researchers realised that a trial that utilised reassurance as its outcome measure would from its outset accept the medical version of what the test was about. As they note, the first quantitative study had conceptualised the test as 'an isolated clinical event with objective benefit flowing from the test itself' (Daly *et al.*, 1992, p. 190).

It was apparent therefore that a different research design that would provide an analysis of the experience of both the cardiologists and the patients when the test was used to diagnose normality was required. Extensive unstructured interviews and the collection of other qualitative data followed. Adopting Strauss's concept of theoretical sampling (Strauss, 1987), subjects were recruited until conceptual categories were saturated and no new categories emerged. The results of this study indicated, among other things, that the reason for having the test done was not, as had been asserted by the doctors, to reassure patients. Instead, the primary reason why the test was undertaken was to comply with the expectations of the referring doctor.

This evaluation of the processes surrounding the ordering and interpretation of a clinical test and its impact on patients revealed results that could not have been elucidated by an RCT. An interesting footnote must also be added, which testifies to the overwhelming hegemony of biomedicine within this field. Bearing in mind the scepticism with which their results might be greeted, these researchers felt it necessary not only to build an account from the interview material that would, in sociological circles, have been deemed adequate, but to convert their interpretation into quantifiable gradings, which could in their turn be verified by a number of independent observers. Perhaps these sorts of additional methodological strategy may be required to convince those who still adhere strictly to traditional epidemiological designs that other approaches may provide additional, or even superior, benefits to an imaginative and yet rigorous assessment of the wide range of disparate healthcare technologies that require evaluation.

Surveillance and control

Individuals or communities?

Epidemiology is the major discipline providing data concerning the extent of health problems in communities and how they differ over time. The focus of these studies is by definition groups, rather than individuals, and one of the objectives is to monitor trends over time in order that control measures may be instituted where necessary. Thus surveillance activities often provide the basis for changes and improvements leading to future healthcare practices.

Although much of nursing involves active participation and intervention in patient care, another important component involves the monitoring of people and their environment. This includes such activities as the regular recording of 'vital signs' in hospitalised patients, weighing babies in the first months of life, testing the urine of pregnant women for protein concentrations and many other similar activities. These monitoring or surveillance activities are designed to ensure that any deviation from what might be considered normal recovery postoperatively, normal postnatal growth, or normal urinary protein concentration is detected early enough for prompt intervention or control measures to be instituted.

These examples draw on nursing practice, which is focused on the individual, but community health and community assessment is important also. Although these latter aspects receive relatively little attention in the training of nurses and midwives, they are integral and almost paramount to health visiting. Ironically, nursing's commitment to the ideology of individualised care may have obscured the importance of how the health of the community may impact on those individuals. Nurses, midwives and health visitors alike need to take note of the context and environment of those individual patients in their care.

Community nursing in the UK is conceptualised as practice that occurs 'in the community' rather than in institutions, but the concept of community relevant to this discussion is more generic. Thus a community might be an antenatal class, a group of drug addicts attending a rehabilitation clinic, a mother and toddler group, an intensive care unit, a residential home for the elderly or a particular family. Definition of the community will depend on the practice setting, the type of healthcare that is provided and the nature of the problems that are usually encountered.

The control and surveillance of health problems in communities is an important component of epidemiology and one well suited to its methods of investigation. Since nursing, midwifery and health visiting all have a community dimension, as defined above, an appreciation and grasp of epidemiological methods will enable all these professions to undertake this aspect of their jobs more effectively. The remainder of this section will examine the principles behind epidemiological surveillance and subsequently provide an example of where surveillance techniques have been used in infection control nursing.

Definitions and principles of surveillance

Although surveillance has probably occurred in some shape or form since the time of Hippocrates, it is only recently that such activities have been formally defined and conceptualised. Several definitions are available. Langmuir (1963, p. 182) defined surveillance as 'continued watchfulness over the distribution and trends of incidence through the systematic collection, consolidation and evaluation of morbidity and mortality reports and other relevant data. Intrinsic in the concept is the regular dissemination of basic data and interpretation, to all who have contributed and all others who need to know'. Another definition, provided by Last in his dictionary of epidemiology (1983, p. 101), describes surveillance as 'ongoing scrutiny, generally using methods distinguished by their practicality, uniformity and frequently their rapidity, rather than complete accuracy. Its main purpose is to detect changes in trend or distribution in order to initiate investigative or control measures'. The first definition pinpoints the main stages in a surveillance programme, while the second provides a more practical aspect and includes the purpose of the exercise. The primary purpose of surveillance is thus to detect new or developing problems rapidly so that they may be controlled, but other secondary purposes or uses may be discerned. These include its value in evaluating control measures, providing information relevant to legal protection claims, raising general awareness and supporting or initiating research programmes (Valenis, 1992).

Surveillance is therefore a multipurpose tool which nurses can utilise, but its purpose will be totally negated if only parts of the process are undertaken. Thus there is simply no value (in fact it is a waste of valuable resources which could be used in other areas) to collect surveillance data that are not regularly analysed, interpreted and disseminated to those who need them. Failure to analyse and evaluate the data that are collected may be construed as unethical, as would any omission to investigate a problem once it has been brought to light by the system.

The sources of information used in any surveillance will vary according to its purpose and setting. Some obvious depots of informa-

Table 6.1 *Sources of information that may be used in surveillance schemes*

- Absentee records
- Inpatient notes
- Nursing kardex
- Pre-employment or on going medical examinations/health checks
- Medical records
- Accident and emergency department records
- Accident logs
- Laboratory records

---

tion are shown in Table 6.1. Sometimes a scheme may be devised using such already available sources, but on other occasions new sources of information and strategies for recording will need to be designed and implemented. Whatever the case, enlisting the participation of those who may be involved from the start of the scheme will pinpoint any operational difficulties and highlight issues that have not been considered. More importantly, ownership of the surveillance scheme and an appreciation of its benefits will ensure that the data collected will achieve much higher reliability, validity and intrinsic worth to the user.

Designing and instituting a surveillance system is far from simple, but unfortunately many schemes have been instigated with little forethought or planning as to their operation or ultimate goals. A useful list of questions that practitioners should address is outlined in Table 6.2.

Although computers have revolutionised the collection of such routine types of data, which are seminal to surveillance activities, there are certain limitations to their use. Pre-eminent is the difficulties that may arise in condensing or coding data into a format suitable for computer entry. In addition, despite the widespread availability of computers many nurses have not had the opportunity to become familiar with their use and this may act as a deterrent either to their cooperation or to the collection of rigorous data. Many professionals are loath to admit to such perceived inadequacies, and without prior training may launch into data collection in a haphazard and unreliable way. Increasing workloads and ever-decreasing staff numbers may also dictate that entry of data on computers for surveillance purposes is seen as a low priority to be completed when other tasks are over. This is usually at the end of the working day, when people are most tired and liable to make errors or take short-cuts.

Table 6.2 *Questions practitioners should pose when contemplating setting up a system of surveillance (modified from Valenis (1992, p. 308))*

- How is a case to be defined and reported?
- What is the source of the information and how accurate is it?
- Who reports the case and by what means?
- How frequently will collation and analysis occur?
- Who will interpret the data and how will this be achieved?
- Who needs the information?
- Who can act on the information?
- How is the scheme to be resourced?
- When and how will the scheme be evaluated?

Although audit and evaluation of nursing and medical practice has now become commonplace, the realisation that activities such as surveillance also require auditing is sometimes forgotten. Whether the surveillance scheme is new or established, a plan for systematically checking various aspects is required, and this normally encompasses two perspectives. Firstly, the everyday administration of the scheme must be monitored. This might include an evaluation of the quality and timeliness of reporting, the reliability of, and time taken to collect the data, and the accuracy of coding if computers are used. Secondly, and of more importance, are global questions concerning the scheme. Are its objectives being met? Were any investigations instigated as a result of the scheme? Might they have been instigated anyway? Was it possible to initiate effective control measures? These are important questions, which should be posed at any time, but in the current phase of financial stringency and professional limitation they are crucial. Such evaluations will underwrite the value of the evidence gleaned from surveillance and allow nurses to make an objective case not only to continue the scheme, but also for any improvements in services which might be indicated. A more detailed account of the setting up of a surveillance system may be found in Chapter 12 of Valenis (1992).

Surveillance and infection control nursing: an example

As noted previously, nurses are already loosely involved in many surveillance activities that are not formally organised and focus on individuals rather than communities. It may be the case that certain of these activities could, with an epidemiological 'imagination', provide more fruitful information on which care practices might be based. Furthermore, armed with the principles of epidemiology nurses will be able to more critically scrutinise existing surveillance practices to determine their validity, reliability and appropriateness. One area where surveillance has a long history is in the recording and control of hospital-acquired infections.

Over thirty years ago the Ministry of Health stated that hospitals should initiate a satisfactory system for ascertaining and recording the clinical evidence of all staphylococcal infections (Ministry of Health, 1959). Since then a variety of approaches to the surveillance of hospital acquired infections (HAI) have been taken in the UK, principally using prevalence and incidence studies (Taylor *et al.*, 1990; Leigh *et al.*, 1990). In 1990 it was reported that 87% of infection control teams collected data concerning the rates of 'alert organisms', i.e. micro-organisms such as methicillin-resistant staphylococci which might cause potential cross-infection problems (Glenister *et al.*, 1990).

Meanwhile, in the USA hospitals have been required since 1974 to collect infection data and produce rates of infection for accreditation. The value of this practice was investigated in the Study on the Efficacy of Nosocomial Infection Control (SENIC), which was undertaken by the Centers for Disease Control (CDC). The results indicated that hospitals with an effective infection control and surveillance programme had reduced the incidence of HAI by 32% in a five-year period. However, total continuous surveillance of infections throughout a hospital is expensive, labour-intensive and not necessarily advisable in terms of cost/benefit. In the UK it is principally infection control nurses who are required to undertake surveillance activities, and on average these nurses cover as many as 2000 beds. Such surveillance work must, however, be accommodated alongside their many other educational, administrative and advisory commitments. A number of selective surveillance methods, such as passive ward notification, temperature and drug chart review and review of patients with known risk factors, have been suggested. In order to determine the effectiveness of these selective methods the Department of Health funded a study to be undertaken by a research nurse based at the Central Public Health Laboratories.

Eight different selective surveillance methods were compared separately with a reference method which aimed to identify all patients and infections in the population under study. The effectiveness of the selective methods was ascertained by determining their specificity and sensitivity (see Chapter 3). In addition, the time taken to undertake the different types of surveillance was recorded. This first stage of the

research indicated that laboratory-based ward surveillance was
most sensitive and time-efficient system for detecting patients w
infections. This system involved the infection control nurse makin
ward visits to follow up all positive microbiology reports identified
by the laboratory. Once on the ward the case records were reviewed
and discussions with nursing staff occurred.

Having identified the method of choice a further study was undertaken to determine the practicalities of implementing such a system in
six District General Hospitals. The method detected 70% of hospital-
acquired infections but only 37% of community-acquired infections.
Although all the infection control nurses were able to operate the
surveillance system successfully, the time taken varied between 3.0
and 6.8 hours/100 beds per week.

These studies exemplify some of the opportunities that epidemiological methods can provide for nursing. A research nurse equipped
with appropriate epidemiological experience was able to manage and
conduct these rigorous studies, which not only provided crucial baseline data concerning the ability of different methods of selective
surveillance to detect infections, but further determined the practicalities of using these methods in the service setting. The results have
provided the objective evidence on which infection control teams may
base their choice of surveillance method, and ensured that hard-
pressed infection control nurses utilise their time in the most efficient
and effective way. Further details of these studies may be found in
Glenister *et al.* (1992, 1993a,b).

Risk, prevention and screening

Epidemiology was defined in Chapter 1 as the study of the distribution
and determinants of disease frequencies in populations. In other
words, it is concerned with questions of where and when disease
occurs, how much disease occurs and the factors that determine these
parameters. For clinical medicine and nursing this may provide the
information through which sickness 'events' may be understood, predicted and interpreted. The concepts of risk and prevention are thus
central to the epidemiological enterprise. How these concepts might
be usefully applied within nursing practice will therefore be evaluated
in this final discussion. The provision of definitions will be followed
by an exploration of risk, screening and prevention through the perspectives of conventional epidemiology. Following this, an alternative
dimension will be discussed which either challenges the fundamental
basis of epidemiological risk and prevention precepts, and/or spot-
lights some of their inherent ethical and moral dimensions.

Conventional accounts

Risk is a term that has a multitude of usages, both vernacular and professional, and thus its meaning is often obscured or confused. Its original usage refers to the probability or likelihood of an event (positive or negative) occurring. Within clinical epidemiology this definition has undergone a subtle (or not so subtle) change, so that according to Fletcher *et al.* (1988, p. 91) risk refers to the probability of an 'untoward' event, and more generally to the likelihood that 'people who are without disease, but are exposed to certain factors (risk factors), will acquire the disease'. Risk factors have been classified in many ways to include those associated with the physical environment (such as toxins and infectious agents), the social environment (such as untoward life events) and the individual (such as behavioural characteristics and genetic dispositions to particular diseases). Texts of clinical epidemiology tend to emphasise the more physical, biochemical or genetic aspects, whereas the emphasis in social epidemiology lies on sociocultural and political factors.

Risk may be classified in three ways:

- **Absolute risk**, which is the simple risk for the whole population and equates with incidence.
- **Relative risk**, which is the ratio of incidence in exposed persons to incidence in non-exposed persons. Relative risk indicates the magnitude of the increased risk derived from exposure. It does not relate to absolute risk, so even if the relative risk of disease following exposure is high, the absolute risk of ever getting the disease might be minuscule.
- **Attributable risk**, which is the incidence of disease in exposed persons minus that in non-exposed persons. It is the excess incidence of disease related to exposure.

For most practitioners and their patients attributable risk is a more meaningful concept, since it indicates the actual probability of disease in those who are exposed. This actual probability may be quite small, even where the relative risk of disease following exposure is high.

In clinical practice, information about risk may be useful in a number of ways. Risk factors may be used to *predict* future occurrence of disease (for example, urethral catheterisation often results in patients acquiring a urinary tract infection); to aid in *diagnosis* (thus a rash in a pregnant woman is not likely to be rubella if she is known to have antibodies to this infection – a case of the absence of a risk factor, non-immunity, aiding diagnosis); and to *prevent* disease by the removal of the risk, as in Snow's classic work on cholera transmission (see Chapter 1).

Some caveats to these uses are however, necessary. The presence of a risk factor does not predict a particular future outcome with certainty – not all patients who are catheterised acquire urinary tract infections and not all smokers get lung cancer. In addition, possible risk factors may be linked or confounded with causal factors; they act as markers to the probability of disease, but importantly their removal does not necessarily imply that the risk of disease will be removed.

Many risk factors are ostensibly obvious both to professionals and the layman. Lying in the sun all day is likely to lead to burnt and blistered skin, and exposure to pollen will lead to hay fever in susceptible individuals. Why then is epidemiology required to investigate risk? While practitioners or lay people are capable of predicting exposure/outcome scenarios such as those above, less obvious relationships are difficult to predict when based on individual experience. Fletcher *et al.* (1988) list six situations when personal experience may be insufficient to establish a relationship between risk and outcome:

- long latency between exposure and outcome
- frequent exposure to the risk factor
- a low incidence of the disease
- small risk of exposure
- common disease
- multiple causes of disease

For chronic diseases in particular, the length of time between exposure to a risk factor and the appearance of disease may be many years. It is unlikely that an individual practitioner would pick this up. Also, where multiple risk factors form part of everyday life it is difficult to recognise the risks that they may represent. Only by studying frequencies of disease amongst populations could these effects be discerned. Again, an individual midwife would find it tricky to predict on personal experience alone the factors that might lead to such diseases as congenital toxoplasmosis when only six to seven cases of this infection are recognised to occur each year in the UK (Hall, 1983). Similarly, if a factor only confers a small risk, then the sample sizes for the comparison of exposed and non-exposed groups need to be very large to observe a difference in disease rates. Many epidemiological studies are working from this basis of where small differences in risk may be discounted through bias or chance. For common diseases with already accepted risk factors, such as heart disease and stroke, discerning new risk factors is difficult. Finally, the problem that many chronic diseases have multiple aetiologies and many risk factors have multiple outcomes obscures the elucidation of relationships between exposure and disease in any particular individual. In all these cases above the techniques of epidemiology are required to provide information drawn from the study of populations. The results of these studies may then be extrapolated to individual patients by individual practitioners.

For medical science the ideal method to investigate risk would be through the use of experiments. For ethical reasons these are not usually conducted, although recent medical history provides several infamous instances. These are, however, exceptions, and traditionally epidemiology investigates risk through quantitative studies principally based on cohort designs. Cohort studies assemble a group of people (the cohort), describe their characteristics (particularly those thought to be related to the outcome in question), and then follow their progress over time to determine who develops the outcome in question. The initial characteristics of those who do and those who do not develop the outcome may then be compared. Further details of this design and some examples of where it has been used in nursing will be found in Chapter 1.

Although risk factor assessment has obvious importance in medicine, there is also a place for it in nursing. Of particular relevance to clinical nursing is the recognition of risk factors that might be influenced by alternative methods of patient management or by strict adherence to established clinical protocols. Nurses are often in the optimum position to question traditional practices which might be changed to the benefit of patients. A knowledge of risk factors may form the basis of these arguments for change or modification.

For example, several studies have demonstrated that the length of time a urethral catheter remains *in situ* is the most important risk factor for the acquisition of bacteriuria (Shapiro *et al.*, 1984; Mulhall *et al.*, 1988). Armed with this knowledge, nurses should strive to ensure that catheters are removed as soon as is feasible and are not left *in situ* for trivial or convenience reasons. Certainly, recent research indicates that the duration of catheterisation for patients who have undergone urological surgery could be safely reduced (Feldstein and Benson, 1988).

Prevention and screening activities also have a basis within a consideration of risk factors. Prevention has been classified at three levels: primary, secondary and tertiary. Primary prevention relates to activities that attempt to stop untoward events appearing at all, for example vaccination programmes or regulations to ensure that blood donations are free from infectious agents such as hepatitis B and C viruses. Secondary prevention aims to detect disease at its early stages when treatment may be instituted to stop the condition from progressing – pap smears to detect pre-malignant cells in the cervix are an example. Tertiary prevention concerns activities that occur once the disease is manifest. The mandate then is to prevent complications or the recurrence of crisis situations. For example, in cases of severe renal disease a kidney transplant may prevent death occurring. The concern of this chapter is with primary and secondary prevention.

Every encounter between health professionals and their clients allows an opportunity for the provision of advice about the primary prevention of ill health. Indeed, *The Health of the Nation* (Department of Health, 1992a) sees health professionals as crucial to the success of its strategy for health, which heavily emphasises the role of preventative measures. For nurses working in hospitals or other institutions in the UK such activities do not loom large, but for others, such as practice nurses, midwives and health visitors, prevention forms a significant component of their remit.

Epidemiology has a considerable role to play here, since any rational programme of health education must be based on communicating the likelihood of ill health associated with certain activities. In other words, it is necessary to know what the **relative** and **attributable** risks associated with exposure to certain activities, such as smoking, drinking alcohol or driving without seat belts, are.

These two expressions of risk encompass quite different concepts (see above) which must also be understood in order that epidemiological evidence may be explained to clients in a meaningful way. Similarly, clients need to be apprised of the potential outcome of any primary preventative measure. For example, parents will wish to know the effectiveness and incidence of side-effects of any proposed vaccines used in childhood immunisation programmes. The well-informed health visitor or school nurse must be able to weigh up the epidemiological evidence related to such issues in order that clients' queries may answered in a factual and honest way. A good grasp of many of the principles that have already been described in this book, such as rates of occurrence, the reliability and validity of measurements, bias and chance, and the factors that affect them, will enable nurses to evaluate the design and methodology of the epidemiological studies that may form the basis of information used in primary prevention.

A prominent strategy in secondary prevention is screening. Screening has been defined as 'the presumptive identification of unrecognised disease or defect by the application of tests, examinations or other procedures that can be applied rapidly and inexpensively to populations' (Valenis, 1992, p. 327). Mass screening of large unse-

Table 6.3 *Criteria for consideration before implementing a screening programme*

- The effect that earlier treatment has on prognosis
- The burden of suffering caused by the condition
- The relative costs and benefits of the programme
- The acceptability of the target population to screening
- The accuracy of the screening test

---

lected populations may occur, such as the screening of new-born babies for phenylketonuria, pregnant women for rhesus factor or adolescent girls for rubella antibodies. Selected mass screening focuses on groups with a known higher risk of certain diseases; for example using mammography to check women with a family history of breast cancer, or chest X-rays for workers with a known exposure to asbestos.

Alongside these mass screenings, individuals now frequently undergo screening during periodic health checks or 'medicals'. Indeed, many health centres and general practitioners are encouraging all their patients to undergo such screening procedures. Many of the screening programmes introduced earlier in this century (such as some of those mentioned above) have had a significant effect in reducing the rates of mortality and morbidity for certain conditions. However, a screening programme should never be instituted before certain criteria have been given careful consideration. These are itemised in Table 6.3.

Obviously there is little advantage, and for the patient there are considerable disadvantages, to screening for a disease for which there is no efficacious treatment, or where early treatment is no more effective than late treatment. The effects of preventative therapy may, however, be very difficult to determine and are only demonstrable through careful large-scale epidemiological studies. Fletcher *et al.* (1988) cite the case of early treatment of breast cancer which required a study lasting 16 years and including 50,000 women to show that this intervention was worthwhile.

A note of caution should be given here concerning lead time – the time between detection of the condition by screening and when it would have been diagnosed usually. Many diseases that result in death are discussed in terms of survival rates. Screening, by detecting a disease earlier, will increase the apparent survival rate over that recorded in persons who are not diagnosed until symptoms appear. Screening might therefore bias the results of a study of the efficacy of early treatment.

From society's point of view it is only economic to screen for diseases that have a relatively high prevalence and which cause a considerable burden of suffering in terms of mortality, morbidity or disability, although any one individual may take a quite different view towards screening. A particular dilemma is posed for those individuals known to be at high risk of a particular condition for which early treatment provides no additional benefit or unknown benefit. Is the peace of mind of periodical negative tests worth the risk of the anxiety if the test is positive? The acceptability of screening tests, both to individuals and to society at large, is an important issue. In contrast with the normal healthcare encounter, screening is usually initiated not by the client but by the healthcare professional or others such as an employer. Indeed, clients may be unaware that they have undergone a screening procedure at all. These issues may pose a number of ethical and moral dilemmas, which will be more thoroughly discussed in the subsequent section.

Finally, the actual screening procedure itself must be carefully scrutinised. Since the prevalence of disease in the asymptomatic population is probably low, the sensitivity of any screening test requires to be high so that these few cases are not missed. Likewise, unless the test is sufficiently specific large numbers of people with false positive results will require further tests incurring additional anxiety, inconvenience and use of health service resources.

Another epidemiological parameter is important in the selection of tests – **predictive value**. The predictive value describes the frequency with which test results represent the correct disease status (present or absent) in those screened. So the positive predictive value of a test represents the probability that people with a positive result actually have the disease in question. The positive predictive value=true positives/true positives+false positives (where a true positive is someone with a positive result and disease present, and a false positive is someone with a positive test result when disease is absent).

Predictive values depend not only on the sensitivity and specificity of a test but also on the prevalence of the disease in the population. As the prevalence of the disease in a population decreases, so does the predictive value of a positive test. This is because even if a test is very specific and therefore results in a small percentage of false positive results, if the majority of the population do not have disease this small percentage could amount to a large number in comparison with the true positives. The positive predictive value as calculated through the equation above will therefore become smaller.

This concept is most easily understood by drawing up a two by two table similar to that in Figure 3.2. and substituting different figures for the prevalence of the disease $(a+c/a+b+c+d)$. Since the prevalence of most diseases is low, predictive values tend to be low, and much time and effort may be spent in following up false positives. This can be avoided as far as possible by focusing screening tests on populations with a higher prevalence of disease. This problem is exemplified by screening for cervical and breast cancers, which are often only taken up by women from populations with a low prevalence of these diseases. This highlights the importance both of targeting groups who are likely to have the highest incidence of disease, and monitoring the programme to ensure that it is indeed this population which responds.

The accuracy of the screening test must also be matched with other more practical criteria. The test must be quick, simple and cheap to perform. It should not require any special preparation by the participants and it should cause them no harm and as little discomfort and inconvenience as possible. The cost of the test will not only be manifest in the test procedure itself and the personnel required to undertake it, but also in the accuracy of the test, which will determine the subsequent number of clients who will require further evaluations.

The criteria discussed above depend on the availability of epidemiological data. Such data include information about the disease, such as its incidence, prevalence and associated mortality; its natural history; the risk factors associated with it; and the safety, sensitivity, specificity and cost of screening tests.

Thus far the opportunities that epidemiological theory and methods may offer to the field of prevention and risk assessment have been considered. The importance of understanding the concepts and technical limitations behind these practices has been outlined in order that new or old procedures may be knowledgeably evaluated. Nurses are often in the position of providing health promotion advice and undertaking such activities as screening or immunisation programmes. A thorough understanding of the underlying principles in this area is essential if nurses are to function effectively as independent practitioners.

There is no doubt that the strategies outlined above are of the utmost importance in maintaining and raising the standards of healthcare in the UK, and much nursing and medical practices are based on them. However, there are some other aspects of prevention in general, and the concept of risk in particular, against which current practices could be usefully considered.

Alternative dimensions

Alongside the well-established uses of epidemiology to prevent ill health, as outlined above, stand some alternative dimensions which require deliberation. Risk has been conceptualised in a number of ways depending on who is using the term. Indeed, the very words used in the language of risk are frequently ambiguous and imprecise – risk factors, risk multipliers, precursors, preconditions – these terms are often left undefined (Hayes, 1992). For epidemiologists, risk exists as a neutral statistical construct referring to the mathematical probability of an event occurring (Hansson, 1989). However, risk is also widely referred to in the discourse of lay people and healthcare professionals. These groups abstract the vocabulary of epidemiological risk and reconstruct this concept in different ways. In contrast with epidemiologists, lay and medical/nursing cultures suffuse risk with a more political and emotional gloss. This may give rise to what Giddens (1984) referred to as the 'double hermeneutic', i.e. the difference in meanings that different groups assign to the same word. The double hermeneutic is ascribed by Nelkin (1985) as exposing the ideological dimensions of risk. The way that concepts such as risk are translated between different groups – lay, nursing, medical – and the conflict over the authority to designate the 'correct translation' is at stake here.

Take the risks associated with childbirth. Obstetricians will justify their preference for high-technology hospital births on the basis that risks in these circumstances are lowered for both mothers and babies. Conversely, midwives use risk to legitimate their opposition to technological births, advocating less intervention. Both groups are implanting the epidemiological concept into their own discourse and in so doing they create risk as a cultural construct rather than a neutral term.

An excellent example of this process is provided by Kaufert and O'Neil (1993) in their account of an epidemiological and anthropological study which examined the impact of evacuating Inuit women from their home towns to meet the official policy of the Canadian Federal Department of Health and Welfare that all births should occur in hospital. The study was developed through an exploration of the three languages of risk – lay, clinical and epidemiological. Data were collected by ethnographical methods which focused on the conversations occurring between lay and professional people at the community meetings called to discuss the general dissatisfaction with the governmental policy. For the Inuit the risks of childbirth were not denied, but rather were accepted as part of the reality of living in the northern part of Canada. Regaining the right to provide an opportunity to give birth locally was a real demand for control over community health, and also a highly symbolic gesture.

In contrast, the clinicians invoked the standard epidemiological language of perinatal and maternal mortality and morbidity, but soon reverted to personal experience to emphasise their point. Thus, rather than grounding their arguments in statistics, as an epidemiologist would have done, clinical risk was compounded from cases of actual or narrowly averted disaster. The fear of postpartum haemorrhage was a leitmotif which kept occurring throughout clinicians' descriptions of birth outside hospital. Birth, blood and death are recognised within anthropology as universally and emotionally powerful themes and 'the idea of seeing a woman bleeding to death and being unable to do anything catches particularly at the medical imagination' (Kaufert and O'Neil, 1993, p. 47). The language of clinical risk was therefore bound up with feelings of personal responsibility and the need to be perceived as competent by others. Risk depended on the speakers, the context in which the conversation occurred, and the historical and political background to the discussion. For Inuit women risk is constructed through community experience. Statistical rates derived through epidemiology lack local validity – the occasional risks of childbirth are a natural part of life. For the clinician, however, risk in childbirth is an ongoing and frightening aspect of clinical life. Both parties failed to grasp the significance of each other's arguments. Ultimately the question concerns who has the power to define risk. As Kaufert and O'Neil (1993, p. 51) conclude, 'Should it be the woman or the physician, the Inuit community or the federal government?'.

This study provides an insight into how the epidemiological concept of risk may be utilised in the healthcare discourse – how neutral statistical concepts may be taken up and transformed into a central cultural construct that will determine how people make sense of their lives. In this sense, risk becomes a hegemonic conceptual tool through which certain 'cultural' agendas are pursued. Traditional epidemiology provides statistical data, which in the example above would include such parameters as the incidence of perinatal mortality, premature birth and Caesarean section. The risks of such events could thereby be calculated for any given population and circumstance.

However, these figures only have meaning in the epidemiological discourse and in relation to other sets of numbers. Healthcare is provided by people and for people, and as such is as much, if not more, a social activity than a scientific one. This is particularly true for nursing, but also for medicine. The ways through which different sets of actors construct risk have significant implications. Epidemiological risk has been hijacked into these other agendas, where it is embodied as a political and moral construct. This dimension of risk becomes particularly pertinent in the context of the primary prevention of ill health through health education, and particularly through health promotion.

As was discussed in the previous section, risk within epidemiology and public health has become synonymous with danger. Certain groups are 'at risk', particular risk factors may enhance any individual's propensity to ill health, and mass media health education campaigns warn of the dangers of certain lifestyles. In fact, today's society is particularly attuned to risks of every kind. As Douglas and Wildavsky (1982, p. 10) note, modern individuals are afraid of 'Nothing much... except the food they eat, the water they drink, the air they breathe, the land they live on and the energy they use'. Much of the healthcare discourse on risk focuses on lifestyle choices and thereby places responsibility and control with the individual. For example, the predominant message in *The Health of the Nation and You* (Department of Health, 1992e) rests on each individual's duty to eat, drink and exercise sensibly. You owe it to yourself!

This individualism is deeply rooted in biomedicine, where the client is seen as deficient and understanding is reconstructed around the problem of the diseased individual body (Crawford, 1977). Naidoo (1986) notes three criticisms to this approach: it denies that health is a social construct; it assumes that free choice exists; and it is not effective within its own terms of reference. There is abundant evidence that ill health and health are socially and culturally constructed (see Chapter 2 for a fuller discussion of this). Free choice may be an option, but again it is often inextricably bound up within a wider politico-economic discourse. Lastly, the third diktat of the individualistic model makes the profound assumption that changes in knowledge lead to changes in behaviour.

Blaxter (1990) in her study of health and lifestyles illustrates the complex relationship that exists between values, attitudes and beliefs, and how these vary in different groups. The potential benefits of health promotion are less than straightforward and exposure to health risks may be involuntary. The relevance and merit of many health education strategies is therefore questionable (Beattie, 1991).

Similarly, Douglas and Calvez (1990) illustrate the complexity of healthcare beliefs and how they affect behaviour in a study of attitudes to the risk of infection with HIV. They note that large sections of the community at risk are impervious to such information. They either 'know' unshakeably that they are immune to risk, or they recognise death as normal and take no steps to avoid it.

The scope of involvement in health education is wide, and all the major 'caring' professions – nursing, medicine, midwifery, health visiting, teaching and social work – claim a stake. In the wider perspective health education is not just about educating lay people about health. It is part of a much wider debate encompassing issues of professional power and political stances and expediencies (Beattie, 1991). Furthermore, the literature on risk acceptance and avoidance in the health domain studiously avoids any discussion of the social context of risk or the political uses to which the risk discourse may be put. As Lupton (1993, p. 428) notes, 'People's fears about risk can be regarded as ways of maintaining social solidarity rather than as reflecting health or environmental concerns. Risk may have less to do with the nature of the danger than the ideological purposes to which concerns about risk may be put'. This is amply demonstrated throughout history where ethnic minorities have been regularly scapegoated when an epidemic broke out. Risk has replaced sin, and lifestyle risk discourse has gained a cultural resonance consonant with the 'desire to explain sickness and death in terms of volition – of acts done, or left undone' (Rosenberg, 1986, p. 50).

There are problems in using epidemiological data produced from population research in individual health risk appraisals (De Friese and Fielding, 1990), and little research has been undertaken into the ethical consequences of such exercises. Quite apart from the documented ineffectiveness of many governmental public information campaigns (Beattie, 1991), such strategies may be coercive and manipulative, playing as they frequently do upon people's emotions, guilts and fears. Victim blaming may also occur. Rodmell and Watt (1986) cite the example of women who are held responsible for the family diet when in reality social and economic forces may render them powerless in this respect. These issues raise important moral and ethical dilemmas for the healthcare professionals charged with promoting health education.

Other prominent primary prevention techniques also cannot solely be evaluated through epidemiological precepts. Turshen (1989) recounts a pertinent tale which illustrates how a seemingly straightforward primary prevention measure – immunisation – became caught up within wider politico-economic issues. In 1976, following the death of a soldier from swine flu virus, the government of the USA mounted an unprecedented campaign to vaccinate every American against this virus. After six months the campaign was terminated. Why was this unprecedented total campaign mounted, and why was it brought to a halt before time? Some unofficial reasons for initiating the programme have been suggested. These include Gerald Ford's desire to be associated with a massive public health effort in election year; the desire of the Centers for Disease Control to deflect any subsequent criticism of unpreparedness; and the desire of the pharmaceutical industry to realise some large and quick profits (Berliner and Salmon, 1976).

Termination occurred when following a survey of the army base where the soldier died the severity of the disease was brought into question, and alongside this it became obvious that the public health services could not logistically handle the campaign alongside their ongoing commitments.

This campaign served therefore to expose two politico-economic features. Firstly, the inability of the public health services to deliver the programme highlighted the absence of an affordable, accessible and comprehensive primary healthcare service in the USA, which might in other countries have fulfilled this public health task. Secondly, the power of the pharmaceutical companies, who not only received $100 million but also had the foresight to ensure that the government met any liabilities claims relating to vaccine use (estimated at $2.64 billion in 1993). This example once again demonstrates some of the less obvious facets of the ways in which epidemiological data may be used or misused. Mass immunisation campaigns must be analysed not only in terms of the science behind the vaccine and its use according to epidemiological principles, but also through the politico-economic context in which they are mounted (Turshen, 1989).

A major strategy in secondary prevention involves the screening of otherwise fit individuals for the presence of symptomless 'disease'. Some of the criteria for screening programmes were discussed above, but one aspect – the ethical and moral dimension of screening – requires further expansion here. Firstly, mass screening may create demands for healthcare that cannot subsequently be met. This is particularly true in non-Western countries, but may also apply to certain groups, such as the elderly, in industrialised societies. For example, there is little to be gained from testing children's eyesight if spectacles are either not available or not affordable.

Secondly, screening can raise anxieties about potential diseases which in fact may never materialise – such is the case with genetic screening for such diseases as cancer. The dilemma here is is it 'better' for people to know that they are at greater risk of a potentially fatal disease or would they rather have never have known and 'taken a chance'? Forewarned they will be able to avail themselves of regular checks for incipient disease (providing these exist), but if early treatment is no better than late treatment, or if there is no effective treatment, then such screening will provoke needless suffering. In the reverse effect, screening may create an undeserved complacency and failure to attend to subsequent signals of deteriorating health.

The other dilemma is of those who are falsely categorised in the 'wrong' group. Such effects are particularly worrisome since, because the prevalence of disease will by definition be low in the screened population, false positive and false negative results are rather likely.

Thirdly, screening may legitimate the creation of stigmatised groups who are labelled 'abnormal'. This is especially relevant where screening occurs in already marginalised groups – for example the screening for sickle cell anaemia among the black population.

Finally, screening may be used by employers or powerful others as a means of social control. Such would be the case in screening for such socially ostracised conditions as AIDS or drug abuse.

These are just a few of the moral and ethical dilemmas that may emerge through the use of screening. Every healthcare professional should be aware of these and any other potential disadvantages to screening before such programmes or individual tests are administered. This is particularly pertinent to the current emphasis on preventative healthcare through regular check-ups or health screens. The implications of such tests must be considered by those administering the tests and discussed fully with clients before, not after, the tests have been undertaken.

This final section has attempted to reveal some of the concerns that a questioning use of epidemiological principles, in preventative healthcare in general and nursing in particular, should bring. Specifically, it has pointed the way towards the appreciation of a broader approach to prevention. This should integrate programmes, policies and other organisational issues and set them against a reality that is economically and politically based. The social and environmental determinants for health must not be ignored through an exclusive focus on an individualistic model. Similarly, prevention should be a shared responsibility that is built up through strategies that recognise the different perspectives that each individual, group or society brings to particular healthcare problems. Epidemiology certainly has a major role to play in these activities, but its assumptions must be continually interrogated in order that optimum use may be made of its opportunities.

Epidemiology is the primary 'feeder' discipline for much of what falls under the rubric of health promotion. It thus frequently sets the agenda for health promotion and frames this agenda within the disease model of health and individualistic medicine. There is a tendency therefore to utilise uncritically the catalogue of disease categories and associated risk factors which are produced through epidemiological methods and directly translate them into health promotion programmes. This may lead to a diversity of campaigns (for example a CHD campaign, a smoking programme or an exercise programme) with essentially similar or overlapping messages. This unsound planning approach results in duplication of effort and information overload.

Together with its reliance on outmoded models of health education, its emphasis on the individual and its narrow view of outcomes, health promotion as based on traditional epidemiology is in grave danger of failing to recognise or affect real human problems. Tannahill (1993) makes the plea for an epidemiology of health to which both medical and social branches would contribute, and which would use new and old methods, subjective and objective measures and a holistic view of the determinants of health. In addition, the importance of the participation of people, and of regarding lay knowledge as not only useful but as valid as scientific information, is gaining ground. This is a vision of epidemiology that nursing can readily align with, espousing as it does many of the concepts and ideologies that underpin the profession.

Some examples of enlightened strategies which take cognisance of these arguments are appearing. For example, South East Thames Regional Health Authority has funded an action-oriented approach to community research (Wainwright, 1993). *Health on the Waterfront* evolved from the informal discussions of health and welfare workers concerning the health problems of people living on the Greenwich and Bexley waterfront. A survey of community attitudes to health was undertaken in an innovative partnership between health sector workers and members of the community. Community development work was synthesised within a framework of lay epidemiology and realised through action-oriented research.

A major concern was to subvert the traditional top-down approach, where members of the community are alienated from the compilation of healthcare data and the subsequent decisions and plans that follow from it. The local population were thus actively involved as equal partners in the research process. Thus, residents decided what should be studied and how the study should proceed. Using ethnographical methods the community development worker identified key inform-ants who were able to pinpoint the main health issues of concern to the local population. These volunteers subsequently played a vital role in both compiling a questionnaire alongside healthcare professionals and administering the survey to the local population.

This collaborative project did not discard traditional epidemiologi-cal principles – for example, random sampling was used to select the participants for the survey, and quantitative measures of prevalence etc. were used to describe the data. However, the framework through which the data were realised was based upon what the target popula-tion considered important. Furthermore, the project was conceived and actioned in true partnership with the community. Such research, based as it is in the reality of people's lives, has a much greater chance not only of revealing pertinent data, but also of identifying strategies through which genuine and achievable changes may be made to improve the health of communities.

The material tackled in the chapter as a whole has covered a wide range of possibilities for the fruitful application of epidemiology in nursing practice. Further examples with particular regard to community and occupational health nursing may be found in Harkness (1995). The areas described here – health technology assessment, surveillance and control, and risk, prevention and screening have been selected as important and representative examples. Hopefully these should go some way to answering the question posed at the outset (Nursing problems – epidemiological answers?). Furthermore, a more critical stance has been adopted in the last section to provoke debate and thought about some of the covert processes that may be ongoing in traditional epidemiological studies. Armed with this questioning framework nursing will be equipped to scrutinise critically both the process and results of epidemiological studies and adopt and adapt them to best meet its clients' needs while recognising its own professional agenda.

CHAPTER SEVEN

Research evaluation and utilisation: the role of epidemiology

The critical assessment of research reports is integral to modern nursing. Not only must practitioners be proficient appraisers of such material, but managers and purchasers (or commissioners) of health services must also be able to recognise significant research findings. Epidemiology offers a set of strategies for reading and organising the literature, particularly quantitative studies, in a systematic way. This chapter will explore how the evaluation of the research literature by nurses might be enhanced, using some of the methods first developed within epidemiology. The first section will reiterate the background to the increasing profile that research is attaining within nursing and outline the major problems that the profession faces in its attempts to use research. Some of the strategies developed within epidemiology for both evaluating and reviewing the literature will then be discussed. The third section will examine the opportunities and constraints afforded to nursing through the adoption of one particular strategy – synthetic research. The chapter will conclude with the enigma of implementation, which will be addressed by exploring some of the issues surrounding research, knowledge and practice

THE IMPORTANCE OF THE RESEARCH LITERATURE

Nursing and research

The Briggs Report (1972) first articulated the need for nursing to base its practice on research, rather than tradition and ritual. Since then, many governmental directives and voices within the profession have reiterated this call (McFarlane, 1984; Department of Health, 1989a, 1993a).

Underlying this movement are two strategies which, although related, have fundamentally different goals. Research-based practice is extolled both as a conduit towards establishing the most effective and efficient method of delivering nursing care, and also as a fundamental prerequisite for the professionalisation of nursing. In terms of this latter goal, it is recognised that a crucial element in establishing the role and status of nursing (or indeed any other occupation) as a profession is a distinct body of knowledge based on research. For nursing, Witz (1994, p. 23) describes this definition and institutional-isation of a unique knowledge base as a credentialist strategy which seeks to both challenge medicine, and to distinguish those who can and those who cannot practice as a nurse. It is thus, in her words, a 'double edged occupational closure strategy'.

Although much official and professional interest has been focused on the need for practice to be founded on rigorous scientific research, the mechanisms through which this might be achieved are less clear and widely debated (Hardey and Mulhall, 1994). Not only are there central dilemmas concerning who should initiate and conduct research in nursing, but questions of how results should be translated for practice, and by whom, also remain unresolved. In addition, with the restructuring of the health service and the changes in nurse education, it is apparent that radical revisions in skill mix may be imminent. The place of healthcare assistants in research or its evaluation has yet to be addressed. It is, however, clear that all qualified nurses will need to demonstrate that their practice is based upon current research. This requirement is both embodied in the UKCC Code of Conduct (UKCC, 1992), and reiterated in policy documents from the Department of Health. For example, Target 9 of *A Vision for the Future* (Department of Health, 1993b, p. vi) states: 'By the end of the year providers should be able to demonstrate at least three areas where clinical practice has changed as a result of research findings'. In consequence, even if they do not conduct research all nurses must be able to access and critically appraise research findings.

Using research in nursing

Although the importance of research evidence in guiding clinical practice is increasingly recognised by both the government and the profession (Department of Health, 1993a,b; UKCC, 1992), there is ample evidence from both the nursing and medical literature that the reality does not match up to the ideal (Walsh and Ford, 1989; Oxman, 1994). There is therefore a growing concern with how research might best be disseminated and implemented. These two terms, and others, such as research 'awareness', 'appreciation', 'literacy' and 'utilisa-tion', are sometimes used interchangeably. This chapter will adopt the following definitions. **Dissemination** refers to the communication of research results to all potential customers – practitioners, educators, managers and other researchers. Research is **used** when it is accessed, read and evaluated with a view to increasing knowledge and understanding. Finally, **implementation** refers to the application of research results in or for practice. Although we are concerned here with all these processes, epidemiology has a particular contribution to make with regard to the dissemination and use of research.

Effective dissemination, use and implementation will depend on many factors related both to individuals and to the organisations in which they work. Implementation will be discussed more fully in the final section of this chapter, while the dissemination and use of research will be addressed here. The effective **use** of research depends on

- a receptive audience
- resources (time, information systems)
- skills

These prerequisites crystallise through a culture in which research is valued and resources are available for studies to be sought out, critically reviewed and their potential for practice recognised. However, it is not enough to read research and apply its results blindly. The formulation of the question, the methodology employed and the interpretation of the results in any study must be carefully scrutinised in the quest for quality research upon which practice may be confidently and ethically based. However, the literature related to healthcare is expanding by 6–7% each year (de Solla Price, 1981) – a volume which threatens to swamp competent researchers in specialised fields, let alone practitioners who may hold more general interests.

In addition, as the ideology of general management gradually pervades nursing, the time available to undertake literature searches and reviews may diminish. Managerial strategies for assessing workload (such as Criteria for Care) utilise estimations of patient dependency that do not necessarily incorporate less overt aspects of nursing, such as the retrieval and evaluation of research articles. More pragmatically, all articles are not of equal importance, and it is necessary to seek out the most valid, reliable and appropriate studies from the great mass produced. All the major healthcare professions are currently addressing these issues, but for nursing particular problems prevail. Three major obstacles lie in the path towards increased research use among nurses:

- the eclecticism of the discipline

- the traditionally poor library and study facilities afforded nursing
- the lack of research evaluation skills among practitioners

Although nursing knowledge is unique and self-determined, it may draw on many disciplines. Thus, in addressing any particular research topic a wide range of different literature may need to be accessed. Take the example of pain, an issue that impinges upon most areas of nursing, midwifery and health visiting. It has long been recognised that pain is not a simple function of the extent of physical damage to the body (Melzack and Wall, 1982). Research into pain has therefore been initiated not only within physiology, pharmacology and medicine, but also by psychologists, sociologists and anthropologists. Furthermore, pain and its alleviation are often of paramount concern in the care of those who are dying. In this respect legal and ethical issues have been raised, widening still further the literature which may need to be consulted.

For medicine, pain is most often conceptualised in terms of physiology and pharmacological interventions, and a review of the 'literature' would therefore be focused and limited to these disciplines. However, nursing holds a more holistic model of pain, and thus recognition of these wider and more varied sources of information would be required. A more radical standpoint would suggest that, as healthcare becomes more integrated and the boundaries between professions blurred, reviews should synthesise all sources of literature in order that practitioners may be provided with a complete overview from which they may select relevant information. One of the difficulties with this approach is the shortage of reviewers skilled across many disciplines who would be competent to undertake this task.

In recognising the wide and varied literature that nurses may need to access, it is ironic that traditionally library and study facilities for nurses have been so poor. Not only has nursing been penalised by a lack of library resources, but the expectation that accessing research should form a legitimate activity within the working day is not yet accepted. Seeking out articles and reading them is regarded as an activity that should occur during off-duty hours. However, without access to major university libraries many nurses remain bereft of the necessary literature through which any comprehensive review might be attained. Basing practice upon research thus becomes a rather arbitrary affair, dependent upon a random array of articles which might become available.

Although this situation is improving, recent commentators (Trevelyan, 1992) have lamented the lack of even basic library facilities for nurses. This lack of resources is compounded by a professional legacy which does not set great store by the written word. Unlike individual academics and ácademic departments, practitioners do not often subscribe to major refereed nursing journals (with the possible exception of the *Nursing Times* and the *Nursing Standard*), or the journals related to other disciplines. Thus a secondary source of research literature is also denied practitioners.

The eclectic nature of nursing also demands a comprehensive knowledge of the location and content of journals, which may range well beyond the familiar confines of 'nursing'. The simple act of identifying the location, content and style of these journals is an added difficulty for nurses. Even within university libraries there are frequently major deficiencies in the range of stock available in the nursing sections. This results from two factors. Firstly, many nursing departments have been recently established in higher education at a time when financial stringency has compelled libraries to reduce their stocks. Secondly, many nursing texts have been written for an audience which underwent training rather than education. The realisation of Project 2000 and the move into higher education has created a demand for higher level texts that meet the demands of these particular students. At present, however, there is a dearth of such books.

To evaluate research studies effectively requires a set of skills that nurse training to date has generally not provided. Indeed, although this problem has been identified as associated with nursing, medicine also suffers a similar deficiency. In order to select the stars from the considerable volume of poor quality material that appears in the healthcare literature, a thorough grasp of research design and methodology is required, for, in a memorable quote, 'too often the "Conclusion" giveth, but the "Materials and Methods" taketh away' (Sackett *et al.*, 1985, p. 290). Many practitioners who trained before the late 1980s have not had the opportunity to attend courses on research methodology. In addition, some Project 2000 courses have failed to reach sufficient depth, or have been taught by lecturers with little real experience of research. There exists then a widespread research illiteracy accompanied by a genuine fear of research and its proponents, methods and claims.

SOME ANSWERS DEVELOPED WITHIN EPIDEMIOLOGY

Two solutions to the problems that practitioners have in accessing and using the research literature have been developed within epidemiology. These are:

- systematic schemes for selecting rigorous studies
- new methods of literature review

Table 7.1 *Reasons for reading journals*

- To check on job advertisements
- To impress colleagues, particularly medical staff
- To keep abreast with political changes in the profession
- To promote a feeling of keeping up to date with developments
- To fulfil the requirements of professional code of conduct
- To enjoy the cartoons or satirical pages
- To learn about new products
- To decide whether to use a new assessment tool
- To enhance critical reading skills
- To find evidence to back up or refute current practice
- To ascertain the risk factors for certain conditions
- To obtain information to impart to others
- To examine the evidence for the effectiveness of certain interventions

Epidemiology's interest in developing methods which enable practitioners to scrutinise and use the research literature more rigorously has been cultivated principally through the development of clinical epidemiology. In particular, the work of the Department of Clinical Epidemiology and Biostatistics at McMaster University in Ontario (1981) (see also Sackett *et al.*, 1991) and that of the University of North Carolina (see Fletcher *et al.*, 1988) stands out. Here much emphasis has been made on attempts to apply the approaches of epidemiology and biostatistics to the practice of medicine; that is, the strategies developed for groups have been adopted for use in individual patients. Although this pioneering work has occurred in medicine there is no reason why nursing should not utilise similar tactics, and indeed it has begun to do so (see below).

Systematic schemes for selecting rigorous articles

There are many and varied reasons for reading research articles. Table 7.1 provides a list that a group of nurses, health visitors and midwives from a community trust in the North of England produced at a recent workshop.

In general, motives for reading may be divided into those related to personal aggrandisement and a desire to maintain abreast of current professional issues and those reasons that more closely embody a commitment to underpin practice with research through a constant appraisal of new or old innovations. It is the latter which are of interest here.

However, before articles may be read they must be retrieved. As noted above, nurses often face a number of difficulties in crossing this, the first hurdle to using research. Assuming access to satisfactory library facilities has been achieved, there are a number of approaches to retrieval that may be adopted. Some involve the use of indexing systems, which are either on-line or more usually now on compact disc systems, such as CD-ROM. For example, MEDLINE, CINAHL (Cumulative Index of Nursing and the Allied Health Literature) and PSYCHLIT may all be accessed through compact disc systems held by the majority of libraries. However, whether the indexes are scanned manually or by computer it is necessary to select keywords to guide the search. The outcome of any search depends crucially on the choice of keywords, and some considerable experience is required to ensure success in this respect.

The above outlines a systematic strategy to accessing the literature, but often a less well-defined route will be followed. Sackett *et al.* (1985) suggest that there are three ways in which the literature may be approached:

- The surveillance approach, where we graze over the literature in search of interesting or relevant items which are set aside for detailed examination later.
- The problem-solving approach, in which the article is read slowly and carefully to provide evidence on which to base practice.
- The exhaustive approach, which approximates to the traditional literature review, and which scans articles of both high and low quality.

Once individual articles have been identified it is necessary to subject them to critical review. Although many articles have been published in the nursing literature concerning critical appraisal (Downs and Newman, 1977; Ward and Fetler, 1979), the approach taken by clinical epidemiology has been rather different. Essentially, nursing has viewed the problem from a research design standpoint. Taking this perspective, articles are appraised according to how close-ly they adhere to a gold standard of design schemata and methods. For researchers (and it is usually they who are penning these articles) this is a feasible approach. However, practitioners are normally provoked into searching the literature as a result of a clinical problem, and the approaches developed within clinical epidemiology may be of greater benefit under these circumstances.

This is not to say that clinical epidemiologists ignore the rigour of design and methodology, but the starting point for their enquiries is firmly based in terms of clinical actions, such as diagnosis, prognosis and treatment. Many articles in the nursing press which describe the process of critically evaluating research reports suggest criteria by which each section of a study (e.g. the abstract, the literature review and the methods) may be appraised. This implies that the entire article must be read and is of scant help to the busy clinician who may quickly become overwhelmed by a mass of literature. Who can say they remain guiltless of assiduously photocopying articles which then gather dust in a tray marked 'Urgent reading'? A more ruthless approach is required.

An initial assessment process will enable the vast majority of articles to be rejected, enabling practitioners to devote sufficient time to those studies that deserve their scrutiny. Occasionally nurses do encounter problems in accessing the literature and finding research which is relevant and applicable to practice; however, more commonly it is information overload rather than scarcity that they face. In the light of this, Sackett *et al.* (1985) have developed a decision tree that enables clinicians to focus attention on those studies which are both valid and applicable to their practice. Figure 7.1 illustrates an adapted version of this decision tree. At first sight it appears to adopt a rather crude methodology. However, expediency must be weighed against the alternative, whereby precious time is wasted wading through poor-quality articles to the detriment of those which are worthwhile. Undoubtedly some high-quality articles may be discarded through this process, but if they are truly excellent it is likely that you will encounter them again and perhaps take a second look.

The title of an article should provide an accurate indication of the content and thrust of the piece, although this is not always the case. However, if the title appears potentially interesting and relevant to your practice, continue.

Although it seems vastly unfair, the track record of authors is an important guide to the *potential* worth of any study. If they have produced useful and rigorous work in the past then there is hope that this paper may be worthwhile also. This approach to weeding out articles is rather unfair to neophyte writers, but just goes to illustrate that it is sometimes worthwhile putting the professor's name in the list of authors!

The quality and format of abstracts or summaries varies widely, and more recently may be strictly prescribed by the requirements of the particular journal. Where this is the case (see, for example, the *British Medical Journal*) quite a lot may be gleaned from the abstract.

The main question here however, is not whether the findings are valid, but if valid, would they be relevant to your practice? Many

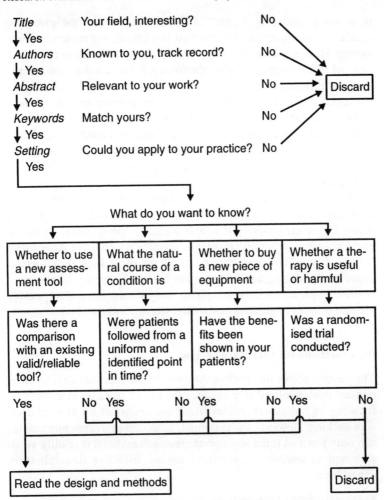

Figure 7.1 *Decision tree for selecting articles (adapted from Sackett et al. (1985, p. 288)).*

journals now list keywords for each article, which may be matched with a list which was compiled (or perhaps held subconsciously) before reading commenced.

Finally, the site and conditions under which the study was conducted should be appraised. If the patients are so dissimilar from your own, or the interventions suggested unlikely to be resourced in your place of work, then you may wish to read no further.

Once these preliminary stages of selection have been undertaken the crucial question is: what do you want to know? Some possible intentions are provided in Figure 7.1. Note that, as with the preceding queries, these questions are couched in clinical, not research, terminology. However, after this stage it is necessary to return to considerations of research design and methodology, for here a decision must be made as to whether an appropriate design was selected to tackle the particular problem raised through the clinical query and, if so, was a valid and reliable methodology pursued. Thus inevitably there is no alternative but to carefully review the design and methods section of the publication. Indeed, having decided to read the paper this should form the core material on which the decision to accept or reject its findings should be based.

Thus the scheme described above does retain some of the features of guides to research appraisal that appear commonly in the nursing press. However, uniquely it adopts a clinical perspective, so that at each stage it is questions relevant to practice which drive the analysis further. For practitioners this provides the most logical and useful approach to reading and scanning the literature. Personal libraries of research information may be built up along similar lines, always using clinical criteria to guide organisation, storage and retrieval.

New methods for literature review

The section above illustrates how some of the methods developed in clinical epidemiology may enhance the use of research in nursing by focusing on individual articles which are important for clinical decision-making. However, the systematic selection of worthwhile articles can only proceed if the appropriate research material is readily available and accessible to practising nurses. Effective **dissemination** depends on:

- the existence of research results
- resources (skilled disseminators, time and money)
- appropriate dissemination vehicles

This section will explore some of the strategies that tackle the problems of dissemination. It will focus on the latter two aspects above, i.e. resources and dissemination vehicles, since these are where epidemiological methods have most impact.

Although some practitioners will always read original articles, there is a widespread and growing conviction that many will need to rely on reviews of the literature to guide their decisions (Williamson *et al.*, 1989). These reviews represent secondary sources of data in that they synthesise the information from several primary research studies. Until recently many of the reviews in books and journals were of the narrative type. Thus an individual (who may or may not be an expert), or rarely a consensus group, would bring together the evidence on the basis of implicit judgement, i.e. opinion. There are some clear dangers here, particularly if the reader is unfamiliar with the topic of concern. Most obviously these traditional narrative reviews are subjective, and rely on idiosyncratic judgements (Pillemer, 1984). Some of the major problems have been summarised by Chalmers (1991) and Cullum (1994a):

- Reviews use only a subset of the available literature and rarely include unpublished material.
- The criteria for inclusion of material are not stated (and usually there are no objective criteria).
- Studies are considered one at a time and the strengths and weaknesses of their design is either not addressed or is discussed *ad hoc*.
- Simplistic or inaccurate conclusions are often drawn.
- The methodology of conducting the review is often omitted – probably because in many cases no formal methodology is adopted.

In addition to these problems associated with traditional unsystematic narrative reviews, several other more general sources of bias have been identified.

Sources of bias in literature studies

Although it has merited little research attention, **publication bias** is recognised by all those involved in the cycle of submitting, selecting, reviewing and editing manuscripts (Dickersin, 1990). The bias manifests as a reluctance to submit or accept articles concerned with research that has failed to demonstrate 'significant' results. 'Negative' studies, especially if they involve a small population sample, have less chance therefore of appearing in print. A current investigation of the publication record for 293 clinical trials funded by the National Institutes of Health in the USA (Dickersin and Min, 1993) indicates that the only factor positively associated with a study's likelihood of publication was the presence of significant results.

Two important observations emerge from this study. Firstly, unpublished trials remained as such because the investigators believed the findings were 'not interesting'. Researchers, rather than editors may therefore be the principle generators of publication bias. Secondly, of 198 trials completed, 93% had been published. This stands in stark contrast to nursing where researchers often fail to publish their results at all – a particular variant of publication bias. For example, a survey by Hicks (1992) reported that although 71% of nurses stated that they had undertaken research only 3% had published their results.

A second source of bias is that associated with the **design and execution** of the individual primary studies that may be incorporated into a review. This may cause particular problems if results are pooled in a quantitative way (see next section) with little regard to the biases that may have existed in the original studies.

Finally, bias may result where there is **incomparability** of patients, interventions or effect measures between the individual studies that are brought together in the review. As an illustration of the last of these, if a midwife was trying to synthesise the results of several studies on the nature of postnatal depression, it would be most important to determine how the factors associated with this condition had been measured in each study included in the review. For example, Beck (1992b), using a qualitative design to investigate the factors associated with postnatal depression reported ten clusters of items which might be relevant to the genesis of this condition. However, she notes that only three of these are included in the Edinburgh Postnatal Depression Scale (Cox *et al.*, 1987), a quantitative tool that is also used to investigate this condition.

As a result of the deficiencies discussed above, the methodology of summarising research in reviews has received some attention in the last ten years. Two important principles have emerged: firstly, that the process by which material is chosen for the review must be made explicit, and secondly that the scientific method is followed more closely. Thus Pillemer (1984, p.29) characterises the structured method of literature review as 'making reviewing practices explicit, and replacing personal decision rules with objective statistical procedures. The reviewer specifies how studies were selected, displays the results summaries on which conclusions are based, and uses integrative techniques, consistent with good statistical practice'. The process of summarising results using this type of structured methodology is termed meta-analysis. Two general approaches to meta-analysis – quantitative summaries and criteria-based or blinded reviews – have been developed within epidemiology. Although these methods have evolved separately, they are not mutually exclusive, and a systematic review often adopts both approaches.

Quantitative summaries

The summarising of results from several studies to obtain one large study with greater statistical power is the format by which meta-analysis is most usually recognised. This technique has been adopted because individual studies often do not include a large enough sample, and therefore run the risk of a Type II statistical error (see Chapter 1). That is, there may be an unacceptably high risk of missing true effects simply because an insufficient number of patients or events were studied. This type of meta-analysis is common in medical research. The debate about serum cholesterol lowering drugs discussed in Chapter 2 provides a good example. The power of meta-analysis has, according to Chalmers (1991), been shown empirically through the demonstration that analyses of past experiments provide a good prediction of future larger studies. He quotes the example of a meta-analysis of four small trials of intra-partum fetal monitoring (Chalmers, 1979), which correctly predicted the results of a larger study (MacDonald *et al.*, 1985). Thus far, nursing has not undertaken many meta-analyses, but some examples are to be found in the work of Waddell (1991) and Goode *et al.* (1991). A more detailed account of the use of meta-analysis in nursing may be found in Abraham *et al.* (1987).

Criteria-based review

In blinded review (or criteria-based meta-analysis) the methods of each individual study included are scrutinised for scientific credibility. Fletcher *et al.* (1988) identify five stages to criteria-based review:

1. Selecting a single clinical question
2. Identifying articles focused on this question
3. Setting criteria according to the nature of the original question
4. Determining how far each study meets the methodological criteria
5. Examining the relationship between the scientific credibility of studies and the conclusions that they draw

It is clear that one of the most important stages in this process, and that most open to interpretation, is the setting of criteria by which studies will be judged. Criteria against which different types of study may be examined have not been universally agreed, although some principles are generally accepted. For example, randomised controlled trials would certainly include criteria that examined the study population (homogeneity, comparability of baseline characteristics); interventions (described in protocol, placebo-controlled); effect measurements (blinded, relevant, adequate follow-up period); and data presentation (intention to treat analysis, description of drop-outs). Other types of design would need to adopt different evaluative criteria.

Criteria may be weighted according to their perceived importance and a sum score may thereby be derived for each study. Some trials may be excluded if certain important criteria are not included. An example of a blinded review of RCTs studying the effects of spinal manipulation for low back and neck pain is provided by Koes *et al.* (1991). Currently, the methodology of blinded reviews remains rather crude, although they do provide some guidance to ascertaining the credibility of the conclusions that are drawn by reviewers.

SYSTEMATIC REVIEWS AND NURSING

Problems with the nursing literature

With the upsurge in interest in the effective dissemination and implementation of research (Department of Health, 1993a), several leading nurses have stressed the importance of synthesising the literature (Hunt, 1987; MacGuire, 1990). The need for critical, systematic reviews in nursing is compelling, for in many respects the nursing literature is more defective than its medical counterpart.

This weakness is manifested in several ways (Mulhall, 1995). The problem of the failure to publish has been mentioned above. In this context Cullum's plea (1994a, p. 50) that 'every effort must be made to locate unpublished as well as published findings, and the so called "grey literature" of conference proceedings...' is apposite. In addition, there has been an abnormally heavy emphasis on papers concerning models and theories of nursing rather than original research. This probably reflects the uncertainties that afflict any discipline during its early development, but again it adds to the dilemma of consolidating evidence upon which practice may be based.

Another concern is that those undertaking nursing research may be drawn from several mother disciplines. In their attempts to address a wide professional audience, research publications may become diluted. Becher (1989) discusses how this phenomenon occurs in other subjects. For example, geography and pharmacy are perceived as having the characteristics of unrestricted knowledge, soft knowledge, divergent communities and applied disciplines. Articles in these two disciplines are often published in journals related to other areas. The journals dedicated to geography and pharmacy tend therefore to be poorly supported and lack prestige (Becher, 1989). Robinson (1993) suggests that nursing follows a similar model. The concerns outlined above suggest that the nursing literature still exhibits weaknesses, both in the reporting of individual studies and in the few narrative reviews that have been published.

Some ways forward

In general, nursing could be strengthened by following the lead of epidemiology and instigating systematic reviews. Some of the sources of bias discussed above might be tackled through a variety of mechanisms. Publication bias could be minimised through the inclusion of unpublished work in systematic reviews; the compilation of registers of ongoing studies; greater credibility being given to large studies (which, whatever their findings, are likely to be published); and more improbably by a journal of negative results!

Bias in individual studies may be addressed through the standardised methodological evaluation described above under *Criteria-based reviews*. Here it is obvious that some further efforts are required to come to a consensus regarding criteria and their respective weightings.

Finally, the bias associated with the incomparability of studies which may be synthesised may be overcome through the use of subgroups within the review, or the imposition of stricter inclusion factors for publications. However, it is apparent that the greatest obstacle to the production of rigorous systematic reviews in nursing may be the quality and availability of original studies. Cullum's systematic review (1994b) of the nursing management of leg ulcers in the community discarded 1600 of the 2000 articles collected and examined as being of such poor quality (according to the criteria of Holm and Llewellyn (1986)) that they were not included in the final review.

The Cochrane Collaboration and the NHS Centre for Reviews and Dissemination

The critical assessment of research reports is essential to research-based practice and the development of nursing knowledge (Mackenzie, 1994). The role that epidemiology may play in enhancing and refining this activity is described in the first part of this chapter. More recent initiatives in this area are based on the premise that busy practitioners will increasingly rely on reviews of primary research to inform their practice. The NHS Research and Development Information Systems Strategy (R and D ISS) provides a framework for these activities and one of its first priorities has been to establish the UK Cochrane Centre and the NHS Centre for Reviews and Dissemination (NHS CRD). These two organisations have been charged with ensuring that up-to-date, critical and relevant reviews of research into the effects of healthcare are made available to practitioners.

The UK Cochrane Centre (named after the late epidemiologist Archie Cochrane) is based in Oxford and modelled on Iain Chalmers' pioneering work on the *Oxford Database of Perinatal Trials* (1992). It is part of an expanding international network of centres which are committed to producing and maintaining systematic reviews – The Cochrane Collaboration. The particular role of the UK Cochrane Centre is 'to collaborate with others to build, maintain and disseminate a database of systematic, up-to-date reviews of randomised controlled trials of health care' (Sheldon and Chalmers, 1994, p. 201). This involves bringing together collaborative review groups composed of individuals who volunteer to prepare and maintain systematic reviews of RCTs for inclusion in The Cochrane Database of Systematic Reviews. Since this material is constantly being updated, the most obvious formats for its dissemination are electronic media. The complete database is therefore distributed on-line and also on CD-ROM, while specialised databases (for example The Pregnancy and Childbirth Database) are available on computer disks. Each Cochrane Centre is also responsible for setting standards governing the reliability of information fed through the database, and for developing new and improved methods of undertaking systematic reviews.

The work of the NHS CRD runs parallel to and complements that of the UK Cochrane Centre. It has three main roles:

- the production of quality reviews
- the dissemination of good research evidence
- the provision of an information and enquiry service

The NHS CRD both commissions and undertakes reviews, which cover the effectiveness of care for specific conditions, the effectiveness of healthcare technologies, and the efficiency of methods of organising the delivery of healthcare. As with the material produced through the Cochrane Collaboration, the emphasis is on the provision of quality reviews that have been produced through internationally accepted guidelines.

Two factors have been instrumental in the development of these centres and their associated work: firstly, the recognition that synthetic research is crucial to the provision of evidence upon which practice may be based, and secondly the realisation that existing methods of review were deficient. Epidemiology and epidemiologists have played a considerable role in the promotion and development of these new techniques for more rigorous review of the literature. Healthcare professionals and their clients should now be in a better position to access and utilise the research evidence relevant to their area of practice.

Potential problems?

Although it cannot be denied that synthetic research has a potentially large and evolving role to play in ensuring the effective utilisation of nursing research, some constraints on its use are apparent. These relate both to intrinsic deficiencies in the current nursing literature, and to the organisational and cultural milieu through which the major initiatives in this area are developing.

The former problem has been discussed more fully above; suffice it to say here that no amount of rigorous methodology in terms of literature review will avail if the range, depth and validity of the individual research studies on which the review is based are not adequate. For many areas of nursing, the research base may be so ill-developed that reviews of the type envisaged are impossible. The disparity of the research base in nursing is a serious concern and has prompted the Department of Health to suggest that 'Each academic department should also seriously consider specialising in a limited number of research fields in which it can clearly establish excellence' (Department of Health, 1993a, p. 15). Systematic reviews have a role to play here in identifying deficiencies and gaps in the knowledge base that require further research.

The latter problem, concerning the cultural milieu in which current initiatives are occurring, arises as a result of the predominantly bioscientific approach that both the Cochrane Collaboration and the NHS CRD adopt, and the fact that these are high-profile government-backed initiatives.

Bioscience, based as it is on positivism and empiricism (see Chapter 6). regards the randomised controlled trial as the apotheosis of 'good' healthcare evaluation (See Chapter 1). It is perceived as the benchmark, or gold standard, against which all other research is judged. Other non-experimental approaches within the positivistic paradigm, such as the observational designs frequently used in epidemiology (see Chapter 1) are deemed second best to the RCT.

In the light of this, the dismissal of other more qualitative research designs and paradigms, such as phenomenology or ethnography, by many natural scientists is understandable. These approaches, it is contended, are worthwhile in their place, but do little to inform about the effectiveness or efficiency of health services. Much of this argument is based on the premise that qualitative research provides subjective rather than objective evidence, and also frequently fails to deliver on that signal characteristic of RCTs – outcome.

Difficulties with the significance and relevance of outcome measurement aside, it should be clear that the process of care is of equal importance to its outcome. In other words, the effectiveness of clinical care cannot solely be judged through its outcome as ascertained by an RCT (see Chapter 6). Furthermore, the view that only research that produces objective evidence is of potential use in systematic reviews is again related to the paradigm in which the natural sciences are functioning, i.e. positivism. Others (Melia, 1982; Duffy, 1985) would contend that many of the processes and phenomena that may be encompassed within health sciences research cannot be investigated through such a paradigm.

Despite some indications that the NHS CRD will use other material it is clear that reviews based on RCTs will predominate, and certainly the ethos that these produce the 'best' evidence for effectiveness prevails. This is clear from the approach taken in early reviews contained in the *Effective Health Care Bulletins* series. For example, the difficulties in interpreting rehabilitation research are discussed thus: 'There are very few well designed and reliable randomised controlled trials that assess the effectiveness of rehabilitation after stroke. Studies typically compare different packages of rehabilitation.... Difficulties in research are compounded by the fact that most patients make some spontaneous improvement.... Given these difficulties the randomised controlled trial *is the best design* [my emphasis] available for assessing the effectiveness of rehabilitation after stroke' (*Effective Health Care Bulletin*, 1992, pp. 3–4). Research grounded in positivism is just one way of 'knowing', and to discard other approaches will not enrich our ultimate knowledge concerning the most effective healthcare that we may offer clients.

Approaches such as ethnography, grounded theory and phenomenology are required to complement the data obtained through quantitative research. These qualitative designs provide information concerning the process of care, which is equally relevant to the determination of effectiveness, as is outcome. By laying bare 'things as they are' (i.e. by taking an interpretist perspective), qualitative designs often reveal and refute assumptions which quantitative research is unable to uncover.

Several examples of the contribution that qualitative designs may make to measuring the effectiveness of healthcare are provided throughout this book (see in particular Chapter 6). Some other studies include Pope's description of the administration of hospital waiting lists (Pope, 1991). This study reports how the day-to-day administration of waiting lists is affected by a variety of factors relating to the office staff and surgeons who process the system. Thus waiting lists were not orderly queues, as perceived by operational managers, but rather less formal systems affected by the structure and staffing of the particular organisation.

Other examples of the use of qualitative research in the evaluation of the effectiveness of healthcare include Silverman's study (1987) of decision-making about the surgical treatment of Down's syndrome children (see Chapter 2) and work by the same author on the effectiveness of different forms of counselling for HIV (Silverman, 1990; Silverman and Perakyla, 1990). A more philosophical analysis of the basis of current health service evaluations and the role of qualitative studies is provided by Dingwall (1992).

If nursing is to make optimum use of these new R and D ISS strategies to produce systematic reviews compatible with its particular models and ideologies, it is clear that the organisation and motivation behind these developments need careful scrutiny. The reorganisation of the health service and the resultant internal market have produced a requirement for health services research of a particular kind. This is much concerned with a narrow interpretation of service – its efficiency, costs, throughput, output etc. It is the evaluation of the service in these terms that will be deemed important by government. Thus the corollary to the statement that the NHS CRD will focus on reviews of specific importance to the NHS (Sheldon and Chalmers, 1994) is 'Who decides what's important?'.

Furthermore, research appropriate to answering these very often economic (in the broadest sense of the word) questions is usually quantitative in nature. The eclecticism of nursing and the paradigms that it embraces indicate that methods for systematic review of the literature will need to include a consideration of qualitative research also (Cullum, 1994a). Methods for systematic integrative review of non-experimental nursing research have been developed (Smith and Stullenbarger, 1991).

A useful synopsis of the philosophy and practice of synthesising qualitative studies is provided by Noblit and Hare (1988). Although synthesising ethnographical accounts has obvious analogies with meta-analysis as discussed so far, these authors adopt a different stance. Arguing that meta-ethnography should be interpretive rather than simply aggregative, they propose the reciprocal translation of key metaphors between individual studies in order to determine the relationships between them. In other words, they are seeking to synthesise understandings across studies, rather than merely aggregating information.

The concept that both qualitative and quantitative research should be included in reviews has been put forward (Light and Pillemer, 1984). It is, however, essential that the hierarchical conceptualisation of research (with RCTs at the top and descriptive and exploratory research at the bottom) which predominates within medicine and epidemiology should be rethought. Research design should rather be viewed as a continuum with positivism at one end and interpretism at the other. Currently, the scientific hegemony, which is operating both generally in the NHS R and D strategy and more specifically in the ISS, may make the achievement of this goal rather remote. The involvement of nurses within these strategies does however provide the opportunity to ensure that the 'continuum' view of research is put forward. However, informed debate of the particular research methods and designs that might best contribute to systematic review can only be achieved from a position of knowledge and with a spirit of flexibility. This will be enhanced by a greater understanding of the opportunities and constraints associated with epidemiology, and an appreciation of the culture in which epidemiologists function.

PROFESSIONALS AND PUBLISHED EVIDENCE – THE ENIGMA OF IMPLEMENTATION

The previous two sections have expanded on how methods developed within epidemiology may enhance the **use** and **dissemination** of research in nursing. Although it is slightly beyond the remit of this text, it is proposed to end the chapter with a consideration of implementation. The reasons for this are twofold. Firstly, it is increasingly recognised both that implementation is crucial to research-based practice, and that existing efforts have been ineffective or non-existent. Research implementation is therefore a major theme in the NHS R and D strategy. Secondly, since strategies to improve implementation are being developed through the R and D ISS, nursing must both take advantage of and contribute to these initiatives.

Effective **implementation** depends on (Mulhall, 1995):

- the availability of appropriate knowledge
- the means to adapt that knowledge to the language and actions of practice
- the opportunity to elicit sustained changes in the way nurses practice

Research and knowledge

It is not possible here to expand in any depth on the subject of nursing knowledge. However, questions concerning epistemology are integral to the evaluation of research and its implementation. Epistemology is the study of knowledge: it asks questions about 'How you know what you know?'. How is knowledge structured? Do all nurses hold the same knowledge and is it structured in the same way? Although these are essentially philosophical debates it is not difficult to understand how they impinge on research implementation. Effective implementation can only be achieved with information about how knowledge, including that obtained through research, is imparted, accumulated and subsequently used by practitioners.

This chapter, indeed this book, has been concerned with the knowledge that may be derived from research. It is important to note, however, that empirical research is not the only source of knowledge. Figure 7.2 outlines some different sources of knowledge which may converge in nursing knowledge, and subsequently be invoked in nursing practice.

Both conceptual knowledge, derived from reflection upon nursing phenomena, and clinical knowledge may complement knowledge gained through research (Schultz and Meleis, 1988). The formulation of clinical knowledge is complex, but probably evolves through experience of both nursing and other related life events, and through intuition. This has implications for implementation, for strategies to integrate research evidence into practice will also need to be consonant with these other sources of knowledge. It will thus be important to understand the different ways in which practitioners call on and structure their knowledge. Research evidence that is discordant with a practitioner's intuitive beliefs is unlikely to be implemented despite the most stringent and strenuous dissemination strategies.

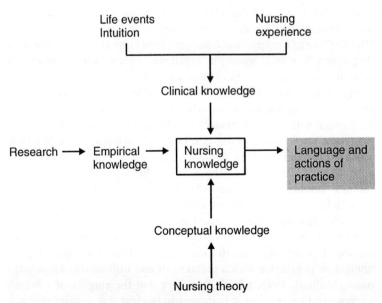

Figure 7.2 *Research, knowledge and practice.*

Research and practice

The activities involved in implementation require not only skills, but also a receptive 'environment'. They depend on effective strategies for introducing research and initiating and managing the appropriate changes in clinical practice. The NHS CRD intends to use a range of methods to promote implementation and to review the evidence of methods which have been effective in influencing behaviour. The Cochrane Collaboration in Effective Professional Practice (CCEP) is also reviewing the effectiveness of implementation strategies across the healthcare professions.

Although certain aspects of research into implementation will be amenable to investigation through quantitative techniques such as surveys, it is crucial that some sensitive and thorough qualitative studies are undertaken also. Implementation strategies must be grounded in an appreciation of the current 'research culture' among practising nurses and their managers. Without this knowledge, valid and well-structured implementation programmes may founder through apathy, indifference or outright opposition.

Even where a synthesis of nursing knowledge as depicted in Figure 7.2 has occurred, implementation will not follow unless this knowledge is transmuted into the language and actions of practice. It is here that the greatest difficulties lie and where many dissemination and implementation programmes have failed through lack of insight into the reasons that may motivate clinicians to practice in the ways that they do. Nurses, midwives and health visitors know that the UKCC *Code of Professional Conduct* (1992) invokes the requirement that research should underpin practice: . 'ensure that no action or omission on [her] part... is detrimental to the interests, condition, or safety of patients...' (UKCC, 1992). 'Action' involving care which research has shown to be harmful, or an 'omission' in becoming acquainted with relevant research would thereby contravene the code. However, diminishing resources, restricted training opportunities, and ever-increasing work demands may dictate that just 'keeping going' is the only option. These are perhaps the stark realities of the new internal market, but other less visible aspects of pragmatism and practice are relevant also.

Much implementation founders as a result of the fundamental disjuncture in the relationship between the discipline and practice of nursing. For 'although the discipline establishes the epistemological domain, it is practice which partakes of and utilises this knowledge base' (Mulhall, 1995, p. 39). It is here that the enigma of research implementation lies, for it is increasingly clear that despite research being available it is not utilised to guide practice (Walsh and Ford, 1989; Oxman, 1994). Why is this?

One reason is that the roles of researcher and carer have different aims and terms of reference (Jelinek, 1992). Researchers are interested in pursuing particular questions with the aim of increasing the theoretical or applied knowledge base. In contrast, practitioners for the most part are attempting to cure or care for people who are (or who may become) sick. This same phenomenon is realised in the different perspectives through which researchers and practitioners approach published information. Clinicians are interested in solving clinical problems, and generally this is the impetus that sends them to the medical or nursing literature. Furthermore, unlike researchers who thrive on the ambiguity and uncertainties revealed through contradictory explanations to problems, practitioners must compromise with pragmatic answers to research questions. Practitioners seek a state of 'optimal ignorance... knowing enough to be effective, but not so much that they become paralysed by uncertainties and ambiguities' (Chrisman and Johnson, 1990, p. 101).

There is no doubt that epidemiology has made a valuable contribution towards solving some of the difficulties inherent in the implementation of research. The accurate identification of valid and reliable research is an obvious prerequisite to implementation. Clinical epidemiology has developed methods for identifying such research and these have been discussed above. In addition, the increasingly sophisticated science of literature review or synthesis was spawned through epidemiology. These initiatives form the basis for much of the current work developing clinical guidelines and standards of practice. These have an undoubted place in increasing the efficiency and effectiveness of health services.

However, the health service is organised and delivered by people. Standardised care may in subtle and not so subtle ways be transformed by the actors involved. Guidelines, even when sensitively produced 'bottom up', are threats to the intuitive aspects of practice which many clinicians set great store by. As Pope and Mays (1994, p. 149), discussing the conflicting voices in health services research, note: 'Despite this 'hard' research evidence,... [RCTs] ...many of the procedures that have been identified as inappropriate or questionable are still used routinely'.

The way forward for implementation must recognise these dilemmas. Critical evaluation skills, systematic reviews, guidelines and standards of practice should form the skeleton of the endeavour. But research derived through different epistemologies and different research approaches must be used to clothe the beast. One solution to relieving the practice/research stalemate is action research. This seeks to change and improve practice through reflection (Schon, 1983). Taking this one step further, Rolfe (1994) has suggested that the explanations of positivistic science and the 'understanding' of qualitative methods such as phenomenology, are insufficient for a nursing research model which must put findings into practice. He thus argues for a research model that incorporates the impetus for change within its methodology. Individualised action research could be realised through reflective practice, which involves a cycle of observation, reflection, conceptualisation and subsequent testing and modification of ideas. This approach to implementation integrates research with practice from the outset and allows practitioners, through their own actions, to become autonomous agents of change.

The two approaches to implementation, discussed here (validation and standardisation modelled on and derived from science, and praxis evolved through individual action) are essentially diametrically opposed both in concept and in practice. At several points in this book it has been suggested that the eclectic nature of nursing might provide the vital links to bring together such opposing viewpoints. Through an appreciation of epidemiology, nursing will be able to grasp the opportunity to umpire this particular dialectic, and ensure that the research, so critical to the provision of effective and appropriate healthcare, is implemented.

Abdellah, F. G. and Levine, E. (1971) *Better Patient Care Through Nursing Research*, Macmillan, New York.

Abel-Smith, B. (1994) *An Introduction to Health: Policy, Planning and Financing*, Longman, London.

Abraham I. L., Schultz, S., Polis, N., Vines, S. W. and Smith, M. C. (1987) Research on research: the meta-analysis of nursing and health research, in *Recent Advances in Nursing: Research Methodology* (ed. M. C. Cahoon), Churchill Livingstone, London, pp. 126–47.

Acheson, R. M., Hall, D. and Aird, L. (1976) *Seminars in Community Medicine. Volume 2: Health Information, Planning and Monitoring*, Oxford University Press, Oxford.

Adams, A., Hardey, M. and Mulhall, A. (1994) Secondary analysis in nursing research, in *Nursing Research: Theory and Practice* (eds. M. Hardey and A. Mulhall), Chapman & Hall, London, pp. 127–44.

Adams, F. (1886) *The Genuine Works of Hippocrates*, William Word, New York.

Alderson, M. R. (1976) Indicators of need, demand and use, in *Seminars in Community Medicine. Volume 2: Health Information, Planning and Monitoring* (eds. R. M. Acheson, D. J. Hall and L. Aird), Oxford University Press, Oxford, pp. 29–40.

Alexander, J. M., Grant, A. M., Campbell, M. J. (1992) Randomised controlled trial of breast shells and Hoffman's exercises for inverted and non-protractile nipples. *British Medical Journal*, **304**, 1030–2.

Allsop, J. (1984) *Health Policy and the National Health Service*, Longman, London.

Andrews, K. (1991) The limitations of randomised controlled trials in rehabilitation research. *Clinical Rehabilitation*, **5**, 5–8.

Annett, H. and Rifkin, S. (1990) *Improving Urban Health*, WHO, Geneva.

Armitage, S. (1990) Research utilisation in practice, *Nurse Education Today*, **10**, 10–15.

Armstrong, D. (1986) The invention of infant mortality. *Sociology of Health and Illness*, **8**, 211–32.

Ashton, J. and Seymour, H. (1991) *The New Public Health*, 3rd edn, Open University Press, Milton Keynes.

Bailar, J. C. (1976) Bailar's laws of data analysis. *Clinical Pharmacology and Therapeutics*, **20**, 113–20.

Bainton, D., Blannin, J. B. and Shepherd, A. M. (1982) Pads and pants for urinary incontinence. *British Medical Journal*, **285**, 419–20.

Bales, V. S. (1983) *Problem Solving for Managers*, US Center for Disease Control, Atlanta.

Ballard, S. and McNamara, R. (1983) Quantifying nursing needs in home health care. *Nursing Research*, **32**, 236–41.

Barker, D. J. P. (1982) *Practical Epidemiology*, Churchill Livingstone, Edinburgh

Beardshaw, V. and Robinson, R. (1990) *New for Old? Prospects for Nursing in the 1990s*, King's Fund Institute, London.

Beattie, A. (1991) Knowledge and control in health promotion: a test case for social policy and social theory, in *The Sociology of the Health Service* (eds. J. Gabe, M. Calnan and M. Bury), Routledge, London, pp. 162–202.

Becher, T. (1989) *Academic Tribes and Territories: Intellectual Enquiry and the Cultures of Disciplines*, Society for Research into Higher Education, Open University, Milton Keynes.

Beck, C. T. (1992b) The lived experience of postpartum depression: a phenomenological study. *Nursing Research*, **41**, 166–70.

Beck, U. (1992a) From industrial society to risk society: questions of survival, social structure and ecological enlightenment. *Theory, Culture and Society*, **9**, 97–123.

Becker, H. S. and Geer, B. (1970) Participant observation and interviewing: a comparison, in *Qualitative Methodology: Firsthand Involvement with the Social World* (ed. W. J. Filstead), Markham Publishing, New York, pp. 133–52.

Benenson, A. S. (1987) Infectious diseases, in *Epidemiology and Health Policy* (eds. S. Levine and M. Lilienfeld), Tavistock Publications, New York, pp. 207–26.

Berliner, H. and Salmon, J. W. (1976) Swine flu the phantom threat. *The Nation*, 25 September, 269–72.

Best, G., Knowles, D. and Mathew, D. (1994) Managing the new NHS: breathing life into the NHS reforms. *British Medical Journal*, **308**, 842–5.

Bevan, A. (1946) *Hansard* (House of Commons), 30 April, col. 52.

Black, Sir Douglas (chair) (1980) *Inequalities in Health. Report of a Research Working Group*. Department of Health and Social Security, London.

Blacklock, N. J. (1986) Catheters and urethral strictures. *British Journal of Urology*, **58**, 475–8.

Blaxter, M. (1990) *Health and Lifestyles*, Tavistock/Routledge, London.

Blaxter, M. and Paterson, E. (1982) *Mothers and Daughters: A Three Generational Study of Health Attitudes and Behaviour*, Heinemann, London.

Bond, J., Atkinson, A., Gregson, B. A. and Newell, D. J. (1989a) Pragmatic and explanatory trials in the evaluation of the experimental National Health Service nursing homes. *Age and Ageing*, **18**, 89–95.

Bond, J., Gregson, B. A., Atkinson, A. and Newell, D. J. (1989b) The implementation of a multicentred randomised controlled trial in the evaluation of experimental National Health Service nursing homes. *Age and Ageing*, **18**, 96–102.

Bor, R., Miller, R. and Johnson, M. (1991) A testing time for doctors: counselling patients before an HIV test. *British Medical Journal*, **303**, 905–7.

Bowling, A. (1991) *Measuring Health. A Review of Quality of Life Measurement Scales*, Open University Press, Milton Keynes.

Brenner, D. J., Steigerwalt, A. G. and Weaver, R. E. (1978) Classification of the Legionnaire's Disease bacterium: An interim report. *Current Microbiology*, **1**, 71–5.

Briggs, A. (1972) *Report of the Committee on Nursing*, Cmnd. 5115, HMSO, London.

Brooks, T. (1992) Total quality management in the NHS. *Health Services Management*, 18 April.

Brown, P. (1987) Popular epidemiology: community response to toxic waste induced disease in Woburn Massachusetts. *Science, Technology and Human Values*, **12**, 78–85.

Brown, P. (1992) Popular epidemiology and toxic waste contamination. *Journal of Health and Social Behaviour*, **33**, 267–81.

Bull, E., Chilton, C. P., Gould, C. A. L. and Sutton, T. M. (1991) Single blind randomised parallel group study of the Bard Biocath Catheter and a silicone elastomer coated catheter. *British Journal of Urology*, **68**, 394–9.

Buss, A. R. (1979) *A Dialectical Psychology*, Invington, New York.

Butler, J. (1992) *Patients, Policies and Politics. Before and After Working for Patients*, Open University Press, Buckingham.

Butler, J. and Vaile, M. (1985) *Health and Health Services: An Introduction to Health Care in Britain*. Routledge & Kegan Paul, London.

Cameron, D. and Jones, I. (1985) An epidemiological and social analysis of the use of alcohol tobacco and other drugs of solace. *Community Medicine*, **7**, 18–29.

Campbell, D. T. and Stanley, J. C. (1963) Experimental and quasi-experimental designs for research, Rand MacNally, College Publishing Co., Chicago.

Carpenter, M. (1977) The new managerialism and professionalism in nursing, in *Health and the Division of Labour* (ed. M. Stacey), Croom Helm, London, pp. 165–93.

Cassell, E. J. (1976) *The Healer's Art: A New Approach to the Doctor–Patient Relationship*, Lipincott, New York.

Chalmers, I. (1979) Randomised trials of fetal monitoring 1973–1977, in *Perinatal Medicine* (eds. O. Thalhammer, K. Baumgarten and A. Pollak), Georg Thieme, Stuttgart, pp. 260–5.

Chalmers, I. (1991) Can meta-analyses be trusted? *The Lancet*, **338**, 1464–5.

Chalmers, I (1992) *Oxford Database of Perinatal Trials*, Version 1.2, Disc Issue 7, Oxford University Press, Oxford.

Chrisman, N. J. and Johnson, T. M. (1990) Clinically applied anthropology, in *Medical Anthropology: Contemporary Theory and Method* (eds. T. M. Johnson and C. F. Sargent), Praeger, New York, pp. 93–113.

Clark, M. and Cullum, N. (1992) Matching patient need for pressure sore prevention with the supply of pressure redistributing mattresses. *Journal of Advanced Nursing*, **17**, 310–16.

Clay, T. (1987) *Nurses: Power and Politics*, Heinemann, London.

Cohen, I. B. (1984) Florence Nightingale. *Scientific American*, **250**, 128–37.

Colgan, M.-P., Dormandy, J. A., Jones, P. W., Schraibman, I. G., Shankin, D. G. and Young, R. A. L. (1990) Oxpentifylline treatment of venous ulcers of the leg. *British Medical Journal*, **300**, 972–5.

Cook, R. L. (1981) Epidemiologic methodology for nurses. *Military Medicine*, **146**, 469–72.

Cook, T. D. and Campbell, D. T. (1979) *Quasi-experimental Design and Analysis Issues for Field Settings*, Houghton Mifflin, Boston.

Cornwall and Isles of Scilly District Health Authority (CISDHA) (1989) *Water Pollution at Lowermoor North Cornwall: Report of the Lowermoor Incident Health Advisory Group* (Chairperson: Professor Dame Barbara Clayton), Cornwall and Isles of Scilly District Health Authority, Truro.

Cox, J. L., Holden, J. M. and Sagovsky, R. (1987) Detection of postnatal depression. Development of the 10 item Edinburgh postnatal depression scale. *British Journal of Psychiatry*, **150**, 782–6.

Cox, T. (1992) *Stress*, 11th edn, Macmillan, London.

Crawford, R. (1977) You are dangerous to your health. The ideology and politics of victim blaming. *International Journal of Health Services*, **7**, 663–80.

Crawford, R. (1984) A cultural account of 'health': control, release and the social body, in *Issues in the Political Economy of Health Care* (ed. J. B. McKinley), Tavistock, London, pp. 60–103.

Crow, R. A., Chapman, R. G., Roe, B. and Wilson, J. (1986) *A Study of Patients with an Indwelling Urethral Catheter and Related Nursing Practice*, Report to the Department of Health, London.

Crowley, P., Elbourne, D., Ashurst, H., Garcia, J., Murphy, D. and Duigan, N. (1991) Delivery in an obstetric birth chair: a randomised controlled trial. *British Journal of Obstetrics and Gynaecology*, **98**, 667–74.

Cullum, N. A. (1994a) Critical reviews of the literature, in *Nursing Research: Theory and Practice* (eds. M. Hardey and A. Mulhall), Chapman & Hall, London, pp. 43–57.

Cullum, N. A. (1994b) *The Nursing Management of Leg Ulcers in the Community. A Critical Review of Research*, Report to the Department of Health, University of Liverpool.

Cullum, N. and Clark, M. (1992) Intrinsic factors associated with pressure sores in elderly people. *Journal of Advanced Nursing*, **17**, 427–31.

Dale, A., Arber, S. and Procter, M. (1988) *Doing Secondary Analysis*, Unwin-Hyman, London.

Daly, J., McDonald, I. O. and Willis, E. (1992) Why don't you ask them?, in *Researching Health Care: Designs, Dilemmas, Disciplines* (eds. J. Daly, I. McDonald and E. Willis), Routledge, London, pp. 189–206.

Daniels, G. (1971) *Science in American Society: A Social History*, Knopf, New York.

Davies, C. (1982) Criticising epidemiology: some notes on the debate. *Radical Community Medicine*, **12**, 6–15.

Dawber, D. R. (1980) *The Framingham Study. The Epidemiology of Athero-schlerotic Disease*. Harvard University Press, Cambridge.

Dealey, C. (1991) The size of the pressure sore problem in a teaching hospital. *Journal of Advanced Nursing*, **16**, 663–70.

De Friese, G. H. and Fielding, J. F. (1990) Health risk appraisal in the 1990s: Opportunities, challenges and expectations. *Annual Review of Public Health*, **11**, 401–18.

Delamothe, T. (1994) Using outcomes research in clinical practice. *British Medical Journal*, **308**, 1583–4.

Department of Clinical Epidemiology and Biostatistics (1981) *Clinical Epidemiology Rounds: How to Read a Clinical Journal*, McMaster University Health Sciences Centre, Ontario.

Department of Health (1989a) *A Strategy for Nursing: A Report of the Steering Committee*, HMSO, London

Department of Health (1989b) *Working for Patients*, Cmnd. 555, HMSO, London.

Department of Health (1989c) *Caring for People: Community Care in the Next Decade and Beyond*. HMSO, London.

Department of Health (1989d) *The Children's Act*, HMSO, London.

Department of Health (1991a) *Research for Health: A Research Development Strategy for the NHS*, Department of Health, London.

Department of Health (1991b) *Water Pollution at Lowermoor North Cornwall: Second Report of the Lowermoor Incident Health Advisory Group* (Chairperson: Professor Dame Barbara Clayton), HMSO, London.

Department of Health (1991c) *The Patient's Charter*, Department of Health, London.

Department of Health (1992a) *The Health of the Nation: A Strategy for Health in England*, HMSO, London.

Department of Health (1992b) *Assessing the Effects of Health Technologies*, Department of Health, London.

Department of Health (1992c) *Public Health Common Data Set. Health of the Nation Baseline Data*, Department of Health, London.

Department of Health (1992d) *Public Health Common Data Set. Health of the Nation Trend Data*, Department of Health, London.

Department of Health (1992e) *The Health of the Nation and You*, HMSO, London.

Department of Health (1993a) *Report of the Taskforce on the Strategy for Research in Nursing, Midwifery and Health Visiting*, Department of Health, London.

Department of Health (1993b) *A Vision for the Future. The Nursing, Midwifery and Health Visiting Contribution to Health and Health Care*, NHSME, Leeds,

Department of Health (1993c) *Targeting Practice: The Contribution of Nurses, Midwives and Health Visitors*, Department of Health, London.

Department of Health (1993d) *Public Health: Responsibilities of the NHS and Roles of Others* (Abraham report), HSG(93)56, Department of Health, London.

Department of Health (1993e) *Public Health Common Data Set. (1993) Including Health of the Nation Indicators*, Department of Health, London.

Department of Health (1993f) *Health Survey for England 1991*. HMSO, London.

Department of Health (1993g) *One Year On: A Report on the Progress of the Health of the Nation*, Department of Health, London.

Department of Health (1993h) *Research for Health*, Department of Health, London.

Department of Health (1994a) *Testing the Vision*, NHSME, Leeds.

Department of Health (1994b) *Health Survey for England 1992*, HMSO, London.

Department of Health (1994c) *R and D Priorities in Relation to the Interface between Primary and Secondary Care*. NHSME, Leeds.

Department of Health and Social Security (1972) *Management Arrangements for the Reorganised Health Service*, HMSO, London.

Department of Health and Social Security (1982) *Steering Group on Health Services Information First Report* (The Körner Report), DHSS, London.

Department of Health and Social Security (1983) *NHS Management Inquiry* (The Griffiths Report), DA(83)38, DHSS, London.

Department of Health and Social Security (1984) *Health Service Management: Implementation of the NHS Management Inquiry Report*, HC(84)13, DHSS, London.

Department of Health and Social Security (1988) *Public Health in England: The Report of the Committee of Inquiry into the Future Development of the Public Health Function* (Chairperson: Sir Donald Acheson), HMSO, London.

Descartes, R. (1649) The passions of the soul, in *Philosophical Works of Descartes* (eds. E. S. Haldane and G. R. T. Ross, transl. 1911), Cambridge University Press, Cambridge, pp. 329–427.

de Solla Price, D. (1981) The development and structure of the biomedical literature, in *Coping with the Biomedical Literature* (ed. K. S. Warren), Praeger, New York.

Dickersin, K. (1990) The existence of publication bias and risk factors for its occurrence. *Journal of the American Medical Association*, **263**, 1385–9.

Dickersin, K. and Min, Y.-I. (1993) NIH clinical trials and publication bias. *The Online Journal of Clinical Trials*, **50**, Agency for Health Care Policy and Research, Rockville, Maryland.

Dingwall, R. (1976) *Aspects of Illness*, Martin Robertson, London.

Dingwall, R. (1992) 'Don't mind him, he's from Barcelona': Qualitative methods in health studies, in *Researching in Health Care. Designs, Dilemmas and Disciplines*, (eds. J. Daly, I. MacDonald and E. Willis), Routledge, London, pp. 161–75.

Dingwall, R., Rafferty, M. and Webster, C. (1988) *An Introduction to the Social History of Nursing*, Routledge, London.

Donabedian, A. (1980) *The Definition of Quality and Approaches to its Assessment*, Health Administration Press, Ann Arbor.

Donaldson, R. J. and Donaldson, L. J. (1993) *Essential Public Health Medicine*, Kluwer Academic Publishers, Lancaster.

Douglas, M. and Calvez, M. (1990) The self as risk taker: A cultural theory of contagion in relation to AIDS. *Sociological Review*, **38**, 445–64.

Douglas, M. and Wildavsky, A. (1982) *Risk and Culture*, Basil Blackwell, Oxford.

Downs, F. S. and Newman, M. A. (1977) *A Source Book of Nursing Research*, F. A. Davis and Co., Philadelphia.

Draper, P. (1991) *Health Through Public Policy: The Greening of Public Health*, Green Print, London.

Draper, P., Best, G. and Dennis, J. (1977) Health and wealth. *Royal Society of Health Journal*, **97**, 121–6.

Duffy, M. (1985) Designing nursing research: the qualitative–quantitative debate. *Journal of Advanced Nursing,* **10**, 225–32.

Dunlop, M. J. (1986) Is a science of caring possible? *Journal of Advanced Nursing,* **11**, 661–70.

Edwards, L. E., Lock, R., Powell, C. and Jones, P. (1983) Post catheterisation urethral strictures: A clinical and experimental study. *British Journal of Urology*, **55**, 53–6.

Effective Health Care Bulletin (1992) *Stroke Rehabilitation*, School of Public Health, University of Leeds, Centre for Health Economics, University of York, Research Unit, Royal College of Physicians.

Eisenberg, L. (1977) Disease and illness: Distinctions between professional and popular ideas of sickness. *Culture, Medicine and Psychiatry*, **1**, 9–23.

Elinson, J. (1974) Towards socio-medical health indicators. *Social Indicators Research*, **1**, 59–71.

Ellis, H. (1992) Conceptions of Care, in *Themes and Perspectives in Nursing* (eds. K. Soothill, C. Henry and K. Kendrick), Chapman & Hall, London. pp. 196–213.

Elston, M. A. (1991) The politics of professional power: medicine in a changing health system, in *The Sociology of the Health Service* (eds. J. Gabe, M. Calnan and M. Bury), Routledge, London, pp. 58–88.

Engel, G. L. (1980) The clinical applications of the biopsychosocial model. *American Journal of Psychiatry*, **137**, 535–44.

Fabrega, H. (1974) *Disease and Social Behaviour: An Interdisciplinary Approach*, MIT Press, Cambridge.

Fabrega, H. and Silver, D. B. (1973) *Illness and Shamanatic Curing in Zinacantan: An Ethnomedical Analysis,* Stanford University Press, Stanford, pp. 218–23.

Farrant, W. and Russell, J. (1985) *Beating Heart Disease: A Case Study in the Production of Health Education Council Publications*, Institute of Education, London.

Feldstein, M. S. and Benson, N. A. (1988) Early catheter removal and reduced length of hospital stay following transurethral prostatectomy: A retrospective analysis of 100 consecutive patients. *Journal of Urology*, **140**, 532–4.

Fletcher, R. H. and Fletcher, S. W. (1979) Clinical research in general medical journals: A thirty year perspective. *New England Journal of Medicine*, **301**, 180–3.

Fletcher, R. H., Fletcher, S. W. and Wagner, E. H. (1988) *Clinical Epidemiology: The Essentials*, Williams and Wilkins, New York.

Flexner, A. (1910) *Medical Education in the United States and Canada*, The Carnegie Foundation for the Advancement of Education, Bulletin 4, New

York.

Flint, C., Poulengeris, P. and Grant, A. (1989) The 'know your midwife scheme': a randomised trial of continuity of care by a team of midwives. *Midwifery*, **5**, 11–16.

Foster, G. M. (1976) Disease aetiologies in non western medical systems. *American Anthropologist*, **78**, 773–81

Foucault, M. (1973) *The Birth of the Clinic*, Tavistock, London.

Foucault, M. (1977) *Discipline and Punish. The Birth of the Prison*, Tavistock, London.

Frankel, S. (1991) Health needs, health care requirements, and the myth of infinite demand. *Lancet*, **337**, 1588–90.

Frankenberg, R. (1980) Medical anthropology and development: a theoretical perspective. *Social Science and Medicine*, **14b**, 197–207.

Frankenberg, R. (1992) The other who is also the same: the relevance of epidemics in space and time for prevention of HIV infection. *International Journal of Health Services*, **22**, 73–86.

Fraser, D. W., Tsai, T. F. and Orenstein, W. (1977) Legionnaire's Disease: Description of an epidemic of pneumonia. *New England Journal of Medicine*, **297**, 1189–97.

Freiman, J. A., Chalmers, T. C., Smith, H., Jr and Kuebler, R. R. (1978) The importance of beta, the Type II error and sample size in the design and interpretation of the randomised controlled trial. *New England Journal of Medicine*, **299**, 690–4.

Friedman, L. M., Furberg, C. D. and DeMets, D. L. (1983) *Fundamentals of Clinical Trials*, Third printing, John Wright, PSG Inc., Boston.

Friedson, E. (1970). *The Profession of Medicine: A Study of the Sociology of Applied Knowledge*, Dodd Mead, New York

Garn, S., Ryan, A. S., Owen, G. and Braham, B. S. (1981) Income matched black–white hemoglobin differences after correction for low transferrin saturations. *American Journal of Clinical Nutrition*, **34**, 1645–7.

Getliffe, K. (1992) *Encrustation of Urinary Catheters in Community Patients*, Unpublished Ph.D. Thesis, University of Surrey, Guildford.

Giddens, A. (1984) *The Constitution of Society: Outline of the Theory of Structuration*, University of California Press, Berkeley.

Glass, N. (1976) Comment on indicators of need demand and use, in *Seminars in Community Medicine. Volume 2: Health Information, Planning and Monitoring* (eds. R. M. Acheson, D. J. Hall and L. Aird), Oxford University Press, Oxford, pp. 41–3.

Glenister, H. (1991) *Surveillance Methods for Hospital Infection*, Unpublished Ph.D. Thesis, University of Surrey, Guildford.

Glenister, H. M., Taylor, L. J., Mackintosh, C. A., Bartlett, C. L. R., Cooke, E. M. and Mulhall, A. B. (1990) Surveillance of hospital infections in the United Kingdom. *Infection Control and Hospital Epidemiology*, **11**, 622–3.

Glenister, H. M., Taylor, L. J., Bartlett, C. L. R., Cooke, E. M., Mackintosh, C. A. and Leigh, D. A. (1992) An 11-month incidence study of infection in wards of a district general hospital. *Journal of Hospital Infection*, **21**,

261–73.

Glenister, H. M., Taylor, L. J., Bartlett, C. L. R., Cooke, E. M. and Mulhall, A. B. (1993a) Introduction of laboratory based ward liaison surveillance of hospital infection into six district general hospitals. *Journal of Hospital Infection*, **25**, 161–72.

Glenister, H. M., Taylor, L. J., Bartlett, C. L. R., Cooke, E. M., Sedgewick, J. A. and Mackintosh, C. A. (1993b) An evaluation of surveillance methods for detecting infections in hospital in-patients. *Journal of Hospital Infection*, **23**, 229–42.

Glick Schiller, N. (1992) What's wrong with this picture? The hegemonic construction of culture in AIDS research in the United States. *Medical Anthropology Quarterly,* **6**, 237–54.

Goldberger, J. and Sydenstricker, E. (1927) Pellagra and the Mississippi flood area. *Public Health Reports*, **42**, 44.

Good, B. and Good, M. J. (1981) The meaning of symptoms: A cultural hermeneutic model for clinical practice, in *The Relevance of Social Science for Medicine* (eds. L. Eisenberg and A. Kleinman), Reidel, Dordrecht, pp. 165–96.

Goode, C. J., Titler, M., Rakel, B., Deniz, S. O., Kleiber, C., Small, S. and Triolo, P. K. (1991) A meta-analysis of effects of heparin flush and saline flush: quality and cost implications. *Nursing Research*, **40**, 324–30.

Gordon, D. R. (1988) Tenacious assumptions in Western medicine, in *Biomedicine Examined* (eds M. Lock and D. R. Gordon), Kluwer Academic Publishers, London, pp. 19–56.

Green, D. G. (1985a) *Which Doctor?*, Institute of Economic Affairs, Research Monograph 40, London.

Green, D. G. (1985b) *Working Class Patients and the Medical Establishment*, Temple Smith/Gower, London.

Habermas, J. (1971) *Knowledge and Human Interests* (transl. J. Shapiro), Beacon, Boston.

Hahn, R. A. (1983) Rethinking illness and disease, *Contributions to Asian Medicine*, **xviii**, 1–22.

Hahn, R. A. and Kleinman, A. (1983) Biomedical practice and anthropological theory. *Annual Reviews of Anthropology*, **12**, 85–93.

Hall, S. M. (1983) Congenital toxoplasmosis in England, Wales and Northern Ireland: some epidemiological problems. *British Medical Journal*, **287**, 453–5.

Ham, C. (1982) *Health Policy in Britain*, Macmillan, London.

Hansson, S. E. (1989) Dimensions of risk. *Risk Analysis*, **9**, 107–12.

Hardy, G. (1981) *William Rathbone and the Early History of District Nursing*, G. W. and A. Hesketh, Ormskirk.

Hardey, M. (1994) Qualitative research and nursing, in *Nursing Research: Theory and Practice* (eds. M. Hardey and A. Mulhall), Chapman & Hall, London, pp. 59–76.

Hardey, M. and Mulhall, A. (1994) *Nursing Research: Theory and Practice*, Chapman & Hall, London.

Harding, J. E., Elbourne, D. R. and Prendville, W. A. (1989) Views of mothers and midwives participating in the Bristol randomised controlled trial of active management of third stage of labour. *Birth*, **16**, 1–6.

Harkness, G. A. (1995) *Epidemiology in Nursing Practice*, Mosby, St Louis.

Harris, A. and Shapiro, J. (1994) Purchasers, professionals and public health. *British Medical Journal*, **308**, 426–7.

Hayes, M. V. (1992) On the epistemology of risk: language, logic and social science. *Social Science and Medicine*, **35**, 401–7.

Haynes, R. B. (1988) Selected principles of the management and setting of priorities of death, disability and suffering in clinical trials. *American Journal of Medical Sciences*, **296**, 364–9.

Headey, B., Homstrom, E. and Wearing, A. (1985) Models of well-being and ill-being. *Health Trends*, **8**, 29–32.

Heginbotham, C. and Ham, C. (1992) *Purchasing Dilemmas*, King's Fund College, London.

Helman, C. (1978) 'Feed a cold starve a fever'. Folk models of infection in an English suburban community, and their relation to medical treatment. *Culture, Medicine and Psychiatry*, **2**, 107–37.

Helman, C. (1990) *Culture, Health and Illness,* Butterworth-Heinemann, London.

Herzlich, C. (1973) *Health and Illness,* Academic Press, London.

Hicks, C. (1992) Of sex and status: a study of the effects of gender and occupation on nurses' evaluations of nursing research. *Journal of Advanced Nursing*, **17**, 1343–9.

Hill, A. B. (1965) The environment and disease. Association and causation. *Proceedings of the Royal Society of Medicine*, **58**, 295–300.

Holm, K. and Llewellyn, J. G. (1986) *Nursing Research for Nursing Practice*, W. B. Saunders, Philadelphia.

Honigsbaum, F. (1979) *The Division in British Medicine,* Kogan Page, London.

Hopkins, A. (1993) What do we mean by appropriate health care? Report of a working group prepared for the Director of Research and Development of the NHS Management Executive. *Quality in Health Care, 2,* 117–23.

Howard-Jones, N. (1974) The scientific background of the International Sanitary Conferences, 1851–1938. *WHO Chronicle*, **28**, 159–71, 229–47, 414–70, 495–508.

Huff, D. (1973) *How to Lie with Statistics*, Penguin, Harmondsworth.

Hulley, S. B. and Cummings, S. R. (1989) *Designing Clinical Research. An Epidemiological Approach*, Williams and Wilkins, Baltimore.

Hunt, M. (1987) The process of translating research findings into practice. *Journal of Advanced Nursing*, **12**, 101–10.

Hunter, D. J. (1980) *Coping with Uncertainties*. John Wiley, Chichester.

Illich, I. (1975) *Medical Nemesis*, Pantheon, New York.

Irvine, J., Miles, I. and Evans, J. (1979) *Demystifying Social Statistics*, Pluto Press, London.

Jacobsen, B. S. and Meininger, J. C. (1985) Designs and methods of published nursing research. *Nursing Research*, **34**, 306–12.

Jelinek, M. (1992) The clinician and the randomised controlled trial, in *Researching Health Care* (eds. J. Daly, I. McDonald and E. Willis), Routledge, London, pp. 76–90.

Jones, K. and Moon, G. (1987) *Health, Disease and Society*, Routledge & Kegan Paul, London.

Kannel, W. B., Dawber, T. R., Glennon, W. E. and Thorne, M. C. (1962) Preliminary report: The determinants of clinical significance of serum cholesterol. *Massachusetts Journal of Medical Technology*, 4, 11–18.

Kaufert, P. A. and O'Neil, J. (1993) Analysis of a dialogue on risks in childbirth, in *Knowledge, Power and Practice. The Anthropology of Medicine in Everyday Life* (eds. S. Lindenbaum and M. Lock), University of California Press, Berkeley, pp. 32–54.

Kelly, G. A. (1966) A brief introduction to personal construct theory, in *Perspectives in Personal Construct Theory* (ed. D. Bannister), Academic Press, London, pp. 1–29.

Kendell, R. E. (1975) *The Role of Diagnosis in Psychiatry*, Blackwell, Oxford.

Kiev, A. (1972) *Transcultural Psychiatry*, Penguin, Harmondsworth.

Klein, R. (1989) *The Politics of the National Health Service*, 2nd edn, Longman, London.

Kleinman, A. (1978). Concepts and models for comparing medical systems as cultural systems. *Social Science and Medicine*, 12, 85–9.

Kleinman, A. (1987) Anthropology and psychiatry. The role of culture in cross-cultural research on illness. *British Journal of Psychiatry*, 151, 447–54.

Kleinman, A., Eisenberg, L. and Good, B. (1978) Culture, illness and care. *Annals of Internal Medicine*, 88, 251–8.

Koes, B. W., Assendelft, W. J. J., Van der Heijden, G. J. M. G., Boulter, L. M. and Knipschild, P. G. (1991) Spinal manipulation and mobilisation for back and neck pain: a blinded review. *British Medical Journal*, 303, 1298–303.

Kuhn, T. (1970) *The Structure of Scientific Revolutions*, University of Chicago Press, Chicago.

Langmuir, A. D. (1963) The surveillance of communicable disease of national importance. *New England Journal of Medicine*, 268, 182–92.

Last, J. (1983) *A Dictionary of Epidemiology*, Oxford University Press, New York.

Last, J. (1987) *Public Health and Human Ecology*, Appleton Lange, East Norwalk CT.

Latour, B. and Woolgar, S. (1979) *Laboratory Life: The Social Construction of Biological Facts*. Sage, Beverly Hills CA.

Leigh, D. A., Emmanuel, F. X. S., Sedgwick, J. and Dean, R. (1990) Post-operative urinary tract and wound infection in women undergoing caesarean section: a comparison of two study periods. *Journal of Hospital Infection*, 15, 107–16.

Leininger, M. (1981) *Caring – An Essential Human Need*, Charles B. Slack, Thorofare NJ.

Levine, S. and Lilienfeld, A. M. (1987) *Epidemiology and Health Policy*,

Tavistock Publications, New York.

Lewis, G. (1993) Some studies of social causes of and cultural response to disease, in *The Anthropology of Disease* (ed. C. G. N. Mascie-Taylor), Oxford University Press, Oxford, pp. 73–124.

Lewis, G., Croft-Jeffreys, C. and David, A. (1990) Are British psychiatrists racist? *British Journal of Psychiatry*, **157**, 410–15.

Light, R. J. and Pillemer, D. B. (1984) *Summing Up: the Science of Reviewing Research,* Harvard University Press, Cambridge MA.

Lilienfeld, A. M. and Lilienfeld, D. E. (1980) *Foundations of Epidemiology*, 2nd edn, Oxford University Press, New York.

Liss, P. E. (1990) *Health Care Need. Meaning and Measurement*, Linkoping University, Sweden.

Llewelyn, H. and Hopkins, A. (1993) *Analysing How We Reach Clinical Decisions*, RCP Publications, London.

Lock, M. and Gordon, D. R. (1988) Relationships between society, culture and biomedicine: An introduction to the essays, in *Biomedicine Examined* (eds. M. Lock and D. R. Gordon), Kluwer Academic Publishers, London, pp. 11–16.

Locker, D. (1983) *Symptoms and Illness*, Tavistock, London.

Lupton, D. (1993) Risk as moral danger: the social and political functions of risk discourse in public health. *International Journal of Health Services*, **23**, 425–35.

MacDonald, D., Grant, A., Sheridan-Pereira, M., Boylan, P. and Chalmers, I. (1985) The Dublin randomised controlled trial of intrapartum fetal heart monitoring. *American Journal of Obstetrics and Gynecology*, **152**, 524–39.

McDonald, I. G., Guyatt, G. H., Gutman, J. M., Jelinek, U. M., Fox, P. and Daly, J. (1988) The contribution of a non-invasive test to clinical care. The impact of echocardiography on diagnosis, management, and patient anxiety. *Journal of Clinical Epidemiology*, **41**, 151–62.

MacFarlane, J. (1984) Foreword, in *The Research Process in Nursing* (ed. D. F. S. Cormack), Blackwell, Oxford, pp. x–xi.

MacGuire, J. (1990) Putting nursing research findings into practice: research utilisation as an aspect of the management of change. *Journal of Advanced Nursing*, **15**, 614–20.

McIver, S. (1991) *Obtaining the Views of Users of the Health Service*. King's Fund Centre for Health and Development, London.

Mackenzie, A. E. (1994) Evaluating ethnography: considerations for analysis. *Journal of Advanced Nursing*, **19**, 774–81.

McKeown, T. (1976) *The Role of Medicine: Dream, Mirage or Nemesis*, Blackwell, Oxford.

MacMahon, B. and Pugh, T. F. (1970) *Epidemiology: Principles and Methods,* Little, Brown and Co, Boston.

Mahomed, K., Grant, A., Ashurst, H. and James, D. (1989) The Southmead perineal suture study. A randomised comparison of suture materials and suturing techniques for repair of perineal trauma. *British Journal of Obstetrics and Gynaecology*, **96**, 1272–80.

Malinowski, B. (1922) *Argonauts of the Western Pacific*, Routledge & Kegan Paul, London.

Marmot, M. G. and McDowell, M. E. (1986) Mortality, decline and widening social inequalities, *Lancet*, **ii**, 274–6.

Martin, P. L. (1972) How preventative is invasive cervical cancer? A community study of preventable factors. *American Journal of Obstetrics and Gynecology*, **113**, 541–8.

Mathews, K. A. and Haynes, S. G. (1986) Type A behaviour pattern and coronary heart disease risk: Update and evaluation. *American Journal of Epidemiology*, **123**, 923–60.

Mausner, J. S. and Kramer, S. (1985) *Epidemiology. An Introductory Text*, W. B. Saunders and Company, Philadelphia.

Maynard, A. (1988) Go easy on the doctor bashing. *Health Service Journal*, **98**, 1068.

Maxwell, R., Hardie, R., Rendall, M., Daly, M., Lawrence, H. and Walton, N. (1983) Seeking quality. *Lancet*, **i**, 45–8.

Melia, K. (1982) 'Tell It As It Is' – Qualitative methodology and nursing research: understanding the nurse's world. *Journal of Advanced Nursing*, **7**, 327–36.

Melzack, R. and Wall, P. (1982) *The Challenge of Pain*, London, Penguin.

Millar, M. A. (1993) The place of research and development in nurse education. *Journal of Advanced Nursing*, **18**, 1039–42.

Ministry of Health (1944) *A National Health Service*, Cmnd. 6502, HMSO, London.

Ministry of Health (1959) *Control of Staphylococcal Infections in Hospitals*, HMSO, London.

Ministry of Health and Scottish Home and Health Department (1966) *Report of the Committee on Senior Nursing Staff* (Chairman Brian Salmon), HMSO, London.

Mischler, E. G. (1981) *Social Contexts of Health, Illness and Patient Care*, Cambridge University Press, Cambridge.

Morsy, S. A. (1978) Sex roles, power and illness in an Egyptian village. *American Ethnologist*, **5**, 137–50.

Morton, R. C. and Hebel, J. R. (1984) *A Study Guide to Epidemiology and Statistics*, Aspen, Rockville.

Mulhall, A. B. (1994) The experimental approach and randomised controlled trials, in *Nursing Research: Theory and Practice* (eds. M. Hardey and A. Mulhall), Chapman & Hall, London, pp. 103–26.

Mulhall, A. B. (1995) *Research: Evaluation and Utilisation*, Distance Learning Centre, South Bank University, London.

Mulhall, A. B., Chapman, R. G. and Crow, R. A. (1988) Bacteriuria during indwelling urethral catheterisation. *Journal of Hospital Infection*, **11**, 253–62.

Mulhall, A. B., Lee, K. and King, S. (1992) Improving nursing practice: the provision of equipment. *International Journal of Nursing Studies*, **29**, 205–11.

Mulkay, M. (1979) *Science and the Sociology of Knowledge*, George Allen & Unwin, London.

Naidoo, J. (1986) Limits to individualism, in *The Politics of Health Promotion* (eds. S. Rodmell and A. Watt), Routledge & Kegan Paul, London, pp. 17–37.

National Advisory Committee on Nutrition Education (NACNE) (1983) *Proposals for Nutritional Guidelines for Health Education in Britain*, Health Education Council, London.

National Health Service and Community Care Act (1991), HMSO, London.

National Health Service Management Executive (1990) *Assessing Health Care Needs*, DHA Project paper, June, NHSME, London.

National Health Service Management Executive (1991) *Moving Forward – Needs, Services, Contracts*. DHA Project paper, March, NHSME, London.

National Health Service Management Executive (1992) *First Steps for the NHS*, NHSME, London.

Navarro, V. (1980) Work, ideology, and science: The case of medicine. *International Journal of Health Services*, **10**, 523–50

Neisser, U. (1966) *Cognitive Psychology*, Appleton-Century-Crofts, New York.

Nelkin, D. (1985) *The Language of Risk*, Sage, Beverly Hills.

Newell, D. J. (1992) Randomised controlled trials in health care research, in *Researching Health Care* (eds. J. Daly, I. McDonald and E. Willis), Routledge, London, pp. 47–61.

Nightingale, F. (1863) *Notes on Hospitals*, Longman, London.

Noblit, G. W. and Hare, R. D. (1988) *Meta-ethnography: Synthesising Qualitative Studies*, Sage, Beverly Hills.

Norton, D., McLaren, R. and Exton Smith, A. N. (1962) *An Investigation of Geriatric Nursing Problems in Hospital*, Churchill Livingstone, London.

Nuffield Institute for Health, Centre for Health economics, Royal College of Physicians (1993) Cholesterol screening and treatment. *Effective Health Care Bulletin*, June, No. 6.

Nyquist, R. and Hawthorn, P. J. (1987) The prevalence of pressure sores in an area health authority. *Journal of Advanced Nursing*, **12**, 183–7.

Oakland, J. S. (1989) *TQM*, Oxford University Press, Oxford.

Office of Health Economics (1982) *Compendium of Statistics 1981*, Office of Health Economics, London.

O'Hare, A. and Walsh, D. (1971) *Irish Psychiatric Hospital Census, 1971*, Medico-social Research Board, Dublin.

Oliver, M. F., Heady, J. A., Morris, J. N. and Cooper, J. (1980) WHO co-operative trial on primary prevention of ischaemic heart disease using clofibrate to lower serum cholesterol: Mortality follow up. *Lancet*, **ii**, 379–89.

Ong, B. N. and Humphris, G. (1994) Prioritising needs with communities. Rapid appraisal methodologies in health, in *Researching the People's Health* (eds. J. Popay and G. Williams), Routledge, London, pp. 58–82.

Oppenheim, A. N. (1984) *Questionnaire Design and Attitude Measurement*, Heinemann, London.

Orem, D. F. F. (1985) *Nursing: Concepts of Practice*, 3rd edn, McGraw-Hill,

New York.

Oxman, A. D. (1994) *No Magic Bullets: A Systematic Review of 102 Trials of Interventions to help Health Care Professionals Deliver Services more Effectively or Efficiently,* Report for North East Thames Regional Health Authority, London.

Parsons, T. (1951) *The Social System,* The Free Press, Glencoe, Illinois.

Pawson, R. (1978) Empiricist explanatory strategies: the case of causal modelling. *Sociological Review,* **26**, 615–40.

Payer, L. (1989) *Medicine and Culture: Notions of Sickness in Britain, USA, France and West Germany,* Gollancz, London.

Perry, A. (1987) Sociology in the curriculum, in *The Curriculum in Nursing Education* (eds. P. Allan and M. Jolley), Croom Helm, Kent, pp. 126–48.

Pill, R. and Stott, N. (1982) Concepts of illness causation and responsibility; some preliminary data from a sample of working class mothers. *Social Science and Medicine,* **20**, 981–91.

Pill, R. and Stott, N. (1985) Preventative procedures and practices among working class women: new data and fresh insights. *Social Science and Medicine,* **21**, 975–83.

Pill, R. and Stott, N. (1987) Development of a measure of potential health behaviour. *Social Science and Medicine,* **24**, 125–34.

Pillemer, D. B. (1984) Conceptual issues in research synthesis. *Journal of Special Education,* **18**, 27–40.

Polit, D. and Hungler, B. (1983) *Nursing Research Principles and Methods,* 2nd edn, Lipincott, Philadelphia.

Pollitt, C. (1992) The struggle for quality: the case of the NHS. *UK Political Studies Association Conference,* Queens University, Belfast, April.

Pollock, K. (1988) On the nature of social stress; Production of a modern mythology. *Social Science and Medicine,* **26**, 381–92.

Pope, C. (1991) Trouble in store: some thoughts on the management of waiting lists. *Sociology of Health and Illness,* **23**, 427–42.

Pope, C. and Mays, N. (1994) Opening the black box: An encounter in the corridor of health services research, in *Nursing Research: Theory and Practice* (eds. M. Hardey and A. Mulhall), Chapman & Hall, London, pp. 145–61.

Posner, T. (1984) Magical elements in orthodox medicine: diabetes as a medical thought system, in *Health and Disease: A Reader* (ed. N. Black), Open University Press, Milton Keynes, pp. 50–6.

Procter, S. (1990) Accountability and nursing. *Nursing Review,* **8**, 15–21.

Ranade, W. (1994) *A Future for the NHS?* Longman, London.

Ransohoff, D. E. and Feinstein, A. R. (1976) Is decision analysis useful in clinical medicine? *Yale Journal of Biological Medicine,* **29**, 165–70.

Ratcliffe, J. W. and Gonzalez del Valle, A. (1988) Rigor in health related research: toward an expanded conceptualisation. *International Journal of Health Services,* **18**, 361–92.

Rhodes, S. (1990) Studying medicine as a cultural system, in *Medical Anthropology. Contemporary Theory and Method* (eds. T. M. Johnson and C. F.

Sargent), Praeger, New York.

Rifkin, S. (1992) Rapid appraisal for health, *Rapid Rural Appraisal Notes*, **July**, pp. 7–12.

Robinson, J. (1993) Problems with paradigms in a caring profession, in *The Art and Science of Nursing* (ed. A. Kitson), Chapman & Hall, London, pp. 72–84.

Rodmell, S. and Watt, A. (1986) *The Politics of Health Promotion*, Routledge & Kegan Paul, London.

Rogers, M. E. (1970) *The Theoretical Basis of Nursing*, Davis, Philadelphia.

Rolfe, G. (1994) Towards a new model of nursing research. *Journal of Advanced Nursing*, **19**, 969–75.

Roper, N., Logan, W. W. and Tierney, A. J. (1990) *The Elements of Nursing. A Model for Nursing Based on a Model of Living*, 3rd edn, Churchill Livingstone, Edinburgh.

Rosenberg, C. E. (1986) Disease and social order in America: Perceptions and expectations. *Millbank Memorial Fund Quarterly*, **64**, 34–55.

Rotter, J. B. (1966) Generalised expectancies for internal versus external control of reinforcement. *Psychological Monographs,* **80** (1).

Russell, I. T., Fell, M., Devlin, H. B., Glass, N. J. and Newell, D. J. (1977) Day case surgery for hernias and haemorrhoids – a clinical, social and economic evaluation. *Lancet*, **i**, 844–7.

Sackett, D. L., Chambers, L. W., MacPherson, A. S., Goldsmith, C. H. and McCaulay, R. G. (1977) The development and application of indices for health. *American Journal of Public Health*, **67**, 423–7.

Sackett, D. L., Haynes, R. B. and Tugwell, P. (1985) *Clinical Epidemiology. A Basic Science for Clinical Medicine*, Little, Brown and Co, Boston.

Sackett, D. L., Haynes, R. B. and Tugwell, P. (1991) *Clinical Epidemiology. A Basic Science for Clinical Medicine*, 2nd edn, Little, Brown and Co, Boston.

Sanders, B. S. (1962) Have morbidity surveys been oversold? *American Journal of Public Health*, **52**, 1648–59.

Sayer, A. (1984) *Method in Social Science: A Realist Approach*, Hutchinson, London.

Scheper-Hughes, N. (1978) Saints, scholars and schizophrenics – madness and badness in western Ireland. *Medical Anthropology*, Summer, part 3, 59–93.

Scheper-Hughes, N. and Lock, M. (1987) The mindful body: A prolegomenon to future work in medical anthropology, *Medical Anthropology Quarterly*, **1**, 6–41.

Schon, D. A. (1983) *The Reflective Practitioner*, Basic Books, New York.

Schultz, P. R. and Meleis, A. I. (1988) Nursing epistemology: traditions, insights, questions. *Image Journal of Nursing Scholarship*, **20**, 217–21

Scott-Samuel, A. (1989) Building the new public health: A public health alliance and a new social epidemiology, in *Readings for a New Public Health* (eds. C. J. Martin and D. V. McQueen), Edinburgh Press, Edinburgh, pp. 29–44.

Seedhouse, D. (1986) *Health: the Foundations of Achievement*, John Wiley, Chichester.

Seedhouse, D. (1994) *Fortress NHS: A Philosophical Review of the National Health Service*, John Wiley & Sons, Chichester.

Shapiro, M., Simchen, E., Izraeli, S. and Sacks, T. G. (1984) A multivariate analysis of risk factors for acquiring bacteriuria in patients with indwelling urinary catheters for longer than 24 hours. *Infection Control*, 5, 525–32.

Sheldon, T. and Chalmers, I. (1994) The UK Cochrane Centre and the NHS Centre for Reviews and Dissemination: Respective roles within the Information Systems Strategy of the NHS R and D Programme, co-ordination and principles underlying collaboration. *Health Economics*, 3, 201–3.

Silverman, D. (1987) *Communication and Medical Practice*, Sage, London, pp. 136–57.

Silverman, D. (1990) The social organisation of counselling, in *AIDS: Individual, Cultural and Policy Dimensions* (eds. P. Aggleton, P. Davies and G. Hart), Falmer, Lewes.

Silverman, D. and Perakyla, A. (1990) AIDS counselling: The interactional organisation of talk about delicate issues. *Sociology of Health and Illness*, 12, 293–318.

Simpson, J. L. and Photopulos, G. (1976) Hereditary aspects of ovarian and testicular neoplasia. *Birth Defects*, 2, 51–60.

Simon, R. (1991) A decade of progress in statistical methodology for clinical trials. *Statistics in Medicine*, 10, 1789–817.

Sleep, J., Grant, A., Garcia, J., Elbourne, D., Spencer, J. and Chalmers, I. (1984) West Berkshire perineal management trial. *British Medical Journal*, 289, 587–90.

Smith, M. C. and Stullenbarger, E. (1991) A prototype for integrative review and meta-analysis of nursing research. *Journal of Advanced Nursing*, 16, 1272–83.

Spencer, P. (1990) *The Riddle of the Sphinx*, Routledge, London.

Spruit, I. P. and Kromhoult, D. (1987) Medical sociology and epidemiology: convergences, divergences and legitimate boundaries. *Social Science and Medicine*, 25, 579–87.

Stacey, M. (1988) *The Sociology of Health and Healing*, Unwin-Hyman, London.

Stainton Rogers, W. (1991) *Explaining Health and Illness*, Harvester Wheatsheaf, London.

Stallones, R. A. (1980) To advance epidemiology. *Annual Review of Public Health*, 1, 69–82.

Stevens, A. and Gabbay, J. (1991) Needs assessment needs assessment. *Health Trends*, 23, 20–3.

Stone, D. (1990) Preventing chronic disease: The dark side of a bright idea, in *Chronic Disease and Disability: Beyond the Acute Medical Model*, Institutes of Medicine, Washington DC, pp. 83–103.

Strauss, A. L. (1987) *Qualitative Analysis for Social Scientists*, Cambridge University Press, Cambridge.

Strong, P. M. and Davis, A. G. (1976) Roles, role formats and medical encounters: A cross cultural analysis of staff client relationships in children's clinics. *Sociological Reviews*, **25**, 775–800.

Strong, P. and Robinson, J. (1990) *The NHS – Under New Management*, Open University Press, Milton Keynes.

Swartz, D., Flamant, R. and Lellouch, J. (1980) *Clinical Trials*, Academic Press, London.

Sydenham, T. (1742) *The Entire Works of Dr Thomas Sydenham* (ed. J. Swan), Edward Cave, London.

Talja, M., Andersson, L. C., Ruutu, M. and Alfthan, O. (1985) Toxicity testing of urinary catheters. *British Journal of Urology*, **57**, 579–84.

Tannahill, A. (1993) Epidemiology and health promotion: a common understanding, in *Health Promotion: Disciplines and Diversity* (eds. R. Bunton and G. Macdonald), 2nd edn, Routledge, London, pp. 86–107.

Taussig, M. (1980) Reification and the consciousness of the patient. *Social Science and Medicine*, **14b**, 3–13.

Taylor, C. (1985) *Human Agency and Language*. Philosophical Papers I, Cambridge University Press, Cambridge.

Taylor, G. W. S., Bannister, G. C. and Calder, S. (1990) Peri-operative wound infection in elective orthopaedic surgery. *Journal of Hospital Infection*, **16**, 241–7.

Temerlin, M. K. (1968) Suggestion effects in psychiatric diagnosis. *Journal of Nervous and Mental Disorders*, **147**, 349–53.

Thomas, C. (1993) Deconstructing concepts of care. *Sociology*, **27**, 649–69.

Thomas, L. (1979) *The Medusa and the Snail*, Viking, New York.

Thomson, G. (1987) *Needs*. Routledge & Kegan Paul, London.

Thunhurst, C. (1991) Information and the public health, in *Health Through Public Policy* (ed. P. Draper), Green Print, London, pp. 118–26.

Trevelyan, J. (1992) Could do better, *Nursing Times*, **88**, 69–72.

Trostle, J. (1986) Early work in anthropology and epidemiology from social medicine to germ theory, 1840 to 1920, in *Anthropology and Epidemiology* (eds. C. R. Janes, R. Stall and S. Gifford), Reidel, Dordrecht, pp. 35–58.

Tuomilehto, J. and Puska, P. (1987) The changing role and legitimate boundaries of epidemiology: Community-based prevention programmes. *Social Science and Medicine*, **25**, 589–98.

Turner, B. S. (1987) *Medical Power and Social Knowledge*, Sage, London.

Turner, B. S. (1992) *Regulating Bodies*, Routledge, London.

Turshen, M. (1989) *The Politics of Public Health*, Zed Books Ltd, London.

Twaddle, A. (1981) Sickness and sickness careers: some implications, in *The Relevance of Social Science for Medicine* (eds. L. Eisenberg and A. Kleinman), Reidel, New York, pp. 111–33.

United Kingdom Central Council for Nursing, Midwifery and Health Visiting (1992) *Code of Professional Conduct*, UKCC, London.

Valabrega, J. P. (1962) *La Relation Therapeutique, Malade et Medicin*, Flammarion, Paris.

Valenis, B. (1992) *Epidemiology and Health Care*, Appleton Laing CT.

Victora, C. G. (1993) What's the denominator? *Lancet*, **342**, 97–9.

Waddell, D. L. (1991) The effects of continuing education on nursing practice:

a meta-analysis. *The Journal of Continuing Education in Nursing*, **22**, 113–18.

Wainwright, D. (1993) *Health on the Waterfront*, Waterfront Health Action Project, London.

Walsh, M. and Ford, P. (1989) *Nursing Rituals: Research and Rational Action*, Butterworth-Heinemann, Oxford.

Ward, M. J. and Fetler, M. E. (1979) Research questions and answers: What guidelines should be followed in critically evaluating research reports? *Nursing Research*, **28**, 120–6.

Watson, J. (1979) *Nursing: The Philosophy and Science of Caring*, Little, Brown and Company, Boston.

Weinstein, M. C., Feineberg, H. V., Elstein, A. S., Frazier, H. S., Neuhauser, D., Neutra, R. R. and McNeil, B. J. (1980) *Clinical Decision Making*, W. B. Saunders, Philadelphia.

White, K. L. (1984) Introduction to health statistics for the year 2000: Patients, primary care, populations and pathology, in *Health Statistics for the Year 2000* (ed. K. Kupka), Statistical Publishing House (for WHO), Budapest, pp. 12–17.

Wilkinson, S. R. (1988) *The Child's World of Illness*, Cambridge University Press, Cambridge.

Williams, G. and Popay, J. (1994a) Lay knowledge and the privilege of experience, in *Challenging Medicine* (eds. J. Gabe, D. Kelleher and G. Williams), Routledge, London, pp. 118–39.

Williams, G. and Popay, J. (1994b) Researching the people's health. Dilemmas and opportunities for social scientists, in *Researching the People's Health* (eds. J. Popay and G. Williams), Routledge, London, pp. 99–114.

Williamson, J. W., German, P. S., Weiss, R., Skinner, E. A. and Bowes, F. (1989) Health science information management and continuing education of physicians. *Annals of Internal Medicine*, **110**, 151–60.

Wilson Barnett, J. and Batehup, L. (1988) *Patient Problems: A Research Base for Nursing Care*, Scutari Press, London.

Witz, A. (1994) The challenge of nursing, in *Challenging Medicine* (eds. J. Gabe, D. Kelleher and G. Williams), Routledge, London.

Woods, N. F. (1980) Women's roles and illness episodes: A prospective study. *Research in Nursing and Health*, **3**, 137–45.

World Health Organisation (1979) *Measurement of Levels of Health*, European Series no. 7, WHO, Copenhagen.

World Health Organisation (1985) *Targets for Health for All, 2000*, World Health Organisation Regional Office for Europe, Copenhagen.

World Health Organisation, Health and Welfare, Canada and Canadian Public Health Association (1986) Ottawa Charter for Health Promotion. *Canadian Journal for Public Health*, **77**, 425–30.

Wright, P. and Treacher, A. (1982) *The Problem of Medical Knowledge: Examining the Social Construction of Medicine*, Edinburgh University Press, Edinburgh.

Young, A. (1980) The discourse on stress and the reproduction of conventional knowledge. *Social Science and Medicine*, **14b**, 133–46.

Young, A. (1982) The anthropologies of illness and sickness. *Annual Reviews of Anthropology*, **11**, 257–85.

Zola, I. (1972) Medicine as an institution of social control, *Sociological Review*, **20**, 487–504.

INDEX